CORE THE
CARE ASS

Edited by

Nigel Conway
Senior Lecturer
Oxford Brookes University

and

Sam Donohue
Oxfordshire Health Care Apprenticeship Co-ordinator
Oxford Radcliffe NHS Trust

Radcliffe Medical Press

Radcliffe Medical Press Ltd
18 Marcham Road
Abingdon
Oxon OX14 1AA
United Kingdom

www.radcliffe-oxford.com
The Radcliffe Medical Press electronic catalogue and online
ordering facility.
Direct sales to anywhere in the world.

British Library Cataloguing in Publication Data

A catalogue record for this book is available from the British Library.

ISBN 1 85775 801 3

Typeset by Aarontype Limited, Easton, Bristol
Printed and bound by TJ International Ltd, Padstow, Cornwall

CONTENTS

PREFACE

The past decade has seen a rapid expansion in the role of health carers and support workers. Alongside this the range of healthcare knowledge and information has escalated. This book sets out to help carers to make sense of this, in a broader context, whilst keeping a clear link to practice.

In this context 'core themes' concern transferable knowledge not specific technical aspects or tasks (such as taking blood pressure). This book is intended to encompass and reflect common aspects of practice that will be used by all health carers, including reflection, the use of evidence to support clinical practice, working in teams, communication, understanding and making use of information, resolving difficult situations, health and safety, developing oneself and being self-directed, legal aspects of care, and lastly, exploring and questioning what is going on around us.

Each of the contributors to this book has been involved directly with the delivery and support of learners undertaking vocational development programmes. There is, therefore, a clear link within the text to the core units of National Vocational Qualifications (NVQ) and the Open College Network units of learning. The Open College Network units were developed by the professional development team within the Oxford Radcliffe NHS Trust and have been used primarily for in-house training programmes with close links to local colleges of further education. This text therefore is suitable for other care providers running local in-house study programmes or education providers offering vocational healthcare courses or healthcare access courses.

Many carers and support staff come to healthcare with a wealth of knowledge and skills gained from previous learning or personal experience. The contributors acknowledge this and aim to build upon it in a way that has a clear link to current healthcare trends.

Each chapter is designed to engage with the reader and contains a number of activities for readers to complete, make notes or answer a specific question. Some of you may be able to complete some of these activities straight away, whereas others may need to find answers to them. Please make use of the spaces provided for your own thoughts and notes.

The chapters also make use of cartoon illustrations and 'top tips'. Top tips identify handy information or 'tips' that may be used to aid learning.

This book will not reduce the need for readers to access other books, articles and journals, or attend teaching or training sessions. However, it should prove a valuable resource and addition to learning.

Each author takes a different approach in terms of writing style. This is intentional and supports the belief of the teams that learning is dynamic and that no one way of information-giving is the only way. Our hope is that the text should prove informative and will help readers to make sense of their role, either now or in the future.

Nigel Conway
August 2003

LIST OF CONTRIBUTORS

Sally Ballard BA (Hons), MA, PGCE, RN
Since registering as a nurse, Sally has worked in clinical, educational and research settings. For two years, she worked as clinical skills tutor for Oxford Brookes University, teaching nursing and operating department practitioners (ODP) students. Sally's lessons on drug calculations led her to consider mathematical ideas and people's understanding of them. She is currently working as a research nurse with the National Blood Service.

Nigel Conway BA (Hons), Cert Ed, FAETC, RODP
Nigel is currently employed as a senior lecturer at Oxford Brookes University. He is a registered operating department practitioner (RODP) and has worked both clinically and educationally in a variety of NHS trusts, private healthcare providers and educational providers. He has been involved with the setting up and delivery of a variety of National Vocational Qualification (NVQ) programmes for different occupational groups.

Billy Count BA
Billy is course team leader and tutor to both the Access to Higher Education (Healthcare) and the Preparation for Diploma courses run at Abingdon and Witney College. Billy has also been involved in writing courses for the access and preparation for diploma programmes. She teaches social sciences related to healthcare, and research and study skills for healthcare students.

Sam Donohue BSc (Hons), Dip HE, RGN, Cert Ed, PG Dip Ed
Sam leads the Oxfordshire Health Care Apprenticeship Programme, an academic and vocational pathway for people wanting to enter professional education. The programme commenced as a route towards a nursing degree but has recently launched a new pre-diploma programme for both nursing and operating department practice. Before moving into education, Sam was ward sister of the Vascular Unit at the Oxford Radcliffe Hospitals NHS Trust.

Claire Evans RGN, FEATC

Claire is a clinical teacher for the Oxfordshire Health Care Apprenticeship Programme. Her nursing background has been in a variety of clinical settings, including acute medicine, diabetes and acute vascular surgery.

Mary Moriarty RMN PGCEA

Mary is currently employed by Oxfordshire Health Care Support Services (OHSS). She has worked clinically for the Oxfordshire Mental Healthcare NHS Trust for many years. She is also the centre co-ordinator for NVQs in Care. Mary facilitates challenging behaviour workshops for a variety of occupational groups in care across Oxfordshire.

Paul Ong MSc, BSc (Hons), RN

Paul is employed as a senior lecturer at Oxford Brookes University. He is a Registered General Nurse and has spent most of his nursing career within gastrointestinal surgery. He has a Postgraduate Diploma in Higher Professional Education and is presently Co-Field Chair for the Adult Nursing Diploma Programme.

Gareth Owens RGN, BSc (Hons), MA Ed, PGCE, Dip Coaching & Mentoring

Currently working as a professional development nurse for the Oxford Radcliffe Hospitals NHS Trust, Gareth has a particular interest in developing policies and educational opportunities that support and develop the role of healthcare assistants. He previously worked as a senior lecturer in the School of Health & Social Care, Oxford Brookes University.

Virginia Playford FAETC, RN

Currently employed as a practice educator within the Oxford Radcliffe Hospitals NHS Trust, Virginia has worked in the health service for 30 years. Her skills and enthusiasm have enabled her to develop her current role and encourage learners of all ages and abilities to improve their skills and qualifications. Virginia has extensive knowledge and experience from many clinical areas. Her current role focuses on education and training within the operating theatre environment which brings her into contact with both vocational and academic learners.

KEY SYMBOLS

 Top tips

 Activities

Chapter 1

PUTTING IT DOWN ON PAPER

Billy Count

INTRODUCTION

Being a student is hard work, and if you are returning to learning it can be especially daunting. Not only have you taken on a new challenge, but you still have all the demands of running a home or holding down a job, or both! This guide is aimed at helping you to study in a smooth, organised manner so that you can use your precious time most effectively. You are given step-by-step help to do something that many people find difficult; you have ideas in your head but now you have to present them to someone else and that means defining them. You may be faced with an essay question, writing a report or you may have been asked to make a presentation on a topic. Whatever it is, you will be faced with the same process of thinking things through, researching and writing; that is where this chapter can help. The focus is on one method of presenting your ideas – writing an essay. These same principles may also be applied to other methods of presenting information.

- Use a loose-leaf folder for your notes so you can re-organise them whenever you want.
- Always write an index card out for any article read.

- Use a computer to draft and write your essays wherever possible.
- Ask a friend to read through your essay and check for any mistakes.

A STEP-BY-STEP GUIDE TO PRESENTING YOUR IDEAS

Compare and contrast two arguments put forward relating to healthy diets, for example eating organic food, eating a balanced low-fat diet or being vegetarian.

When you are faced with an essay question, it is easy to panic, your mind goes blank and your first thought is *'No way! I can't do this!'* Well, you can! Take a deep breath and try it using this guide.

MINDMAP

 Write down everything that comes into your head about healthy diets:

- low fat/high fibre
- vegetarian
- vitamins (now you carry on . . .).
-
-

HEADINGS

Now try and put the notes you have made under a few headings. For example, you might have headings for 'Healthy', 'Unhealthy', 'Medical advice', 'Principles about eating food' (organic, vegetarian, etc.).

RE-READ THE QUESTION

Now you have your headings, read the question again. You are moving on to essay planning so it is vital that you are answering the question that has been set and not a question in your head.

DECIDE THE ARGUMENTS

Decide the arguments you are going to concentrate on. This question asks you to pick two. Other questions may ask you to take a position using only one argument, for example ' "Too much television is bad for you." Do you agree or disagree?'

Now you have chosen your arguments, look at your headings and link them to the arguments you are going to use. For example:

Vegetarian	Low-fat balanced diet
• Principle: kind to animals	• Recommended medically
• Lots of fresh fruit and vegetables	

RESEARCH YOUR IDEAS

Right, so far you have been jotting down your own ideas based on your general knowledge. Now is the time to do some research. There are two main sources: your library and the internet.

Library

If you can go to a college, work or hospital library you will have access to a wider range of referenced work, journals and books. A public library may not be so useful. Referenced work will give details of where any statement made in a book or article may be checked. (It is *essential* that your essay is referenced and this is discussed later.) You will probably find a list of references at the end of the book or journal or at the end of each chapter; in this book the references are at the end of each chapter.

Libraries are all organised according to subject matter. Different libraries will have different systems so the first thing to do is *make a friend of the librarian*. Do not be afraid to go in and ask for help. If you explain what you are looking for, the librarian will show you where to look and may well make some helpful suggestions.

The internet

There is lots of information on the internet – the trick is deciding what is reliable and what is rubbish. Remember that anyone can set up a website and the article that is assuring you that the most healthy diet consists of chocolate, fried eggs and melon balls may not have been written by a qualified nutritionist!

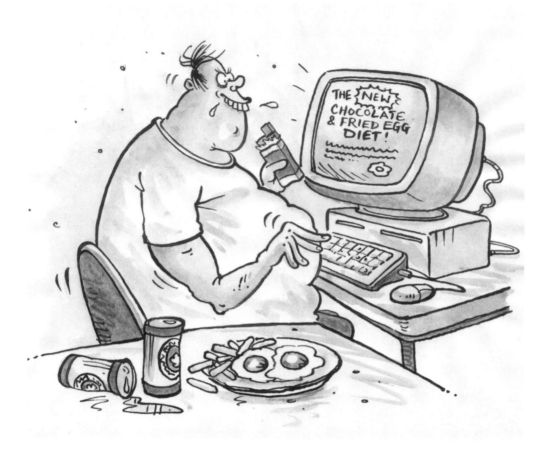

Check who has produced the website. If it is a recognised name, such as the Department of Health, Joseph Rowntree Foundation or Greenpeace, the information on the site should be useable. Because information taken from the internet has this question mark hanging over it a good suggestion is that *no more than half your information should come from this source.*

OK, you have a pile of books, a handful of professional journals and half a tree's worth of computer printouts. Now what do you do?

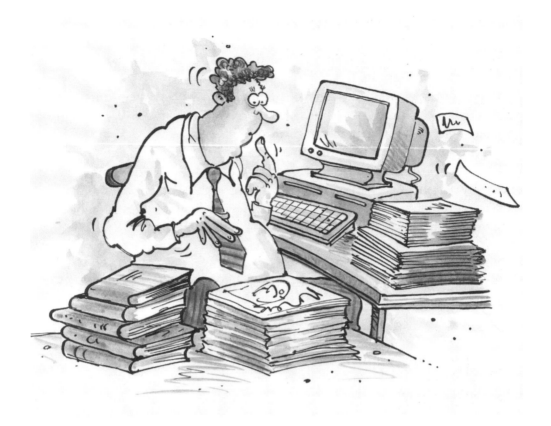

SORTING YOUR EVIDENCE

Start by checking your books and journals. *When were they published?* Unless they contain the original piece of research, the very first time the idea was ever thought of, they should be less than 10 years old.

Imagine you find four books about the food combining diet, one was written by Dr Hay in 1935. Dr Hay was the first person to ever talk about food combining so his work is *seminal* (think of semen, the seed of an idea). You can keep that book because seminal is good, you are getting the original ideas rather than something second-hand and possibly slightly biased. Two books were published in the 1980s – no good; there might have been some new findings, changing scientific opinion, since then. The other book was published just last year, it is really up to date and tells you what *current* thinking about the food combining diet is – great! Keep hold of this one.

Now let us look at the pile of journals. The same rule applies, only current research (less than 10 years old) unless it is seminal. Journals have lots of articles in them so instead of looking at titles of books you are looking at the contents page. If you are lucky, the library will have an index to the articles in a set of journals, so instead of going through each one, you could just look up 'food combining' or 'Hay' in the Index.

By now you have reduced your research pile to two books and perhaps two journals. One book is seminal, the other book and the articles are all current. Now let us see if the internet sources are useful.

By using a search engine, you have already made sure that the articles are relevant, but *who wrote them?* Be ruthless, throw out anything you think might be written by a crank, or anything that seems to be making claims and not backing them up. Internet sources can be referenced too; if they are, this is a good sign that the information is reliable.

MAKING MORE NOTES AND RECORDING YOUR RESOURCES

Don't waste any of your hard work. Get into the habit of always *indexing your resources.* Have a set of index cards and an index card file. Always make notes on a card for each article you look at, *even* if you are not going to use it for this essay, it may well be useful in the future.

On the front of the card:

- Put the full reference (saves time when you are writing your essay).
- The library reference (so you can find it easily another time).
- Where you can find it (printout/photocopy filed in ... or book bought/ 24-hour loan, etc.).

On the back of the card put:

- A summary of what the article says.
- Any strengths and weaknesses?
- Any other comments?

Now unless you are a superhero, you are probably dreading all this reading. Relax! You do not have to read every single word! Use indexes, contents, section headings and summaries to find the topic you are looking for. Once you have narrowed your search to a chapter, for example, you can let your eye drift over the page until you find the key words you are looking for. As soon as you have found the relevant phrase or word, check back through the previous section or paragraph to make sure that this really is the first time the topic is introduced. Once you are certain you have found the beginning, read it in detail.

Gathering infomation

Find three long newspaper articles. Decide what the article is about – the headline will help. Decide which key words or phrase you are looking for. Scan the articles as described above. Time yourself.

Now you have got the information, how are you going to use it in your essay? You cannot just copy it all out. The first thing you need to do is make notes. How do you decide what the important points are? When you take notes, they should be organised into *key points* and *supporting evidence*.

 Do your homework

Watch an episode of your favourite soap/TV programme.

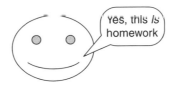

Now imagine you are sitting having a *quick* drink with a friend. Your friend asks what happened on the TV programme last night. Write down what you would tell your friend.

You have just picked out the important or *key points* of the episode, the things your friend needs to know. The same method works if you are reading an academic article. If a friend asked you what the article was all about, you would not repeat it word for word, you would pick out the important bits that explain the message of the text.

Have you ever read one of those articles that pick out the best cars, washing machines or holiday destinations? The writers do not just say the best place for a family to go on holiday is Bournemouth, they *support the statement* by saying that the beach is safe and sandy, accommodation is plentiful and cheap, there are plenty of things to do if it is raining, etc.

What holiday destination would you recommend for a honeymoon or a young family? Give at least two reasons why you are recommending each destination.

- _____ for a honeymoon because:
  - _
  - _
- _____ for a young family because:
  - _
  - _

You have just written down the *supporting evidence* for your statements, this is what you need to look for when you are making notes. The book written by Dr Hay may contain a statement that says something like:

It is bad to combine proteins and carbohydrates together.

This would be a *key point*, now you need to check out why Dr Hay is saying that. Perhaps he would say something like:

They are digested differently. Proteins are only digested by stomach acids, it can take up to three hours to break the food down; carbohydrates are digested in the alkaline environment of the intestines. (Holford, 1997)

This is the *supporting evidence*, now you can add in the conclusion that Dr Hay made, that your digestive system works more efficiently if you only eat one type of food at a time.

So you now have the information from your books, journals and the internet for one argument. Now do the same for the other argument. Remember the question? *Read it again* just to make sure. You are asked to compare and contrast two arguments.

THE ESSAY PLAN

Introduction
Sets out your intentions and *defines* the key terms, for example:

> This essay will examine two arguments of what is a healthy diet: a vegetarian diet compared and contrasted with Dr Hay's food combining diet. Following on from the comparison of diets a conclusion will be reached and presented. A healthy diet is defined as one that meets the nutritional needs of the individual. A vegetarian diet excludes at least fish and animal products; it may also exclude animal byproducts, such as eggs. Dr Hay's food combining diet is . . .

Body
Presents your main arguments.

For your plan you may want to use two columns so you can look at the two arguments clearly. You have been asked to compare (look at the similarities) and contrast (look at the differences) between the two arguments. That means you *do not* write everything about one topic *and then* everything about the other and hope that your tutor will pick out the points you should have made. You *do* go through them point by point, making it very clear where the two arguments have points in common and where they differ, for example:

> Vegetarians and Dr Hay aim to have a healthy diet, however, the difference is that . . .

 There are some important points to note:

- Always put information into your own words *or* put points into 'quotation marks'.
- Always reference your work (*see below*).
- Never pretend that someone else's work is your own (that would be plagiarism or academic stealing).
- Make your points briefly but clearly, do not ____ out anything vital.
- For each point you make, have at least one piece of evidence to back up what you are saying.

Conclusion

Your conclusion, you have examined both arguments in depth, which one do you agree with and why? *Do not* say that, given the evidence above, you agree with X and leave it there, you must make it clear why you are in favour of X.

The conclusion is the most important part of your essay. So far, you have been demonstrating your research abilities, now you need to show that you can take the information you have found, think about it and assess it. Does it make sense? Is it relevant? Is there a counter-argument? Is it logical or is there a flaw? Is the argument based on fact? Is there research to back it up? Imagine you are in the pub and someone at the bar starts spouting out all the arguments put forward by Dr Hay, is there a point where you could (if you could get a word in edge-ways!) say *'Yes, but what about . . .'*?

This is called *critically evaluating* the information. Remember, when something is written in a book, or found on the internet, it might still be complete rubbish! It is your job to try and pick holes in it! An article that vaguely mentions 'studies supporting these findings', for example, should be slated. You are looking for *evidence-based* writing. Lack of references to back up assertions is an immediate point of criticism because you have no way of judging how reliable the information is.

Where details of research are given, check that the numbers used are *big enough to generalise* those findings to the rest of us. A report that states, '20% of boys lose their virginity by age 13' sounds shocking, but less so when you find out that only five teenagers were interviewed. A large sample, such as the British Crime Survey (www.homeoffice.gov.uk) that interviews thousands of citizens, would be far more believable.

Beware of bias, different writers write from their own viewpoints. Seminal works get you closest to the original piece of research but even then read carefully because the researcher may have been biased! Perhaps the researcher was out to prove a pet theory. Be aware that the further away from an original piece of research you are, the more chance there is for distortion to creep in (Hartley, 2001).

ESSAY DRAFT

Your plan is set out in notes, now you need to draft your essay. If you use a computer you will be able to edit again and again rather than re-writing several times. You have done the hardest bit in the essay plan, writing it should be easy! Set your work out in paragraphs remembering to *be clear* at each stage, use phrases such as 'the advantages are', 'these theories differ in that ...', 'the similarities are ...'. You are showing your understanding of what is involved *and* you are making it easier for your tutor to mark your work – always a good idea!

Each time you back up a point you have made with supporting evidence you need to *cite your reference*. This means you have to put in the name of the person who wrote the article you have read, or the name of the person who conducted a particular experiment. Follow this with the date the article or research was published. If you refer to the author directly, cite your reference like this:

Smith and Jones (2001) state that grass is green because ... .

If you refer to the work indirectly, cite your reference like this:

Grass is green because ... (Smith and Jones, 2001)

Try to write out any information you use in your own words, this shows your understanding, and *always acknowledge your source*. Published work is precious to academics and not acknowledging your source would be seen as stealing someone else's ideas or hard work, it is known as plagiarism and is taken extremely seriously.

At the end of your essay, you should list your references in *alphabetical order* using the Harvard referencing system. Follow the simplified guide overleaf (Table 1.1).

THE FINAL PIECE OF WORK

It is downhill all the way now! You have got your draft written out. Just follow this checklist to the finishing line:

- Check again: have you answered the question?
- If you were given one, have you kept to the word count?
- Check your word count in Microsoft Word by going to File > Properties > Statistics.
- Could anyone else read your handwriting?
- Check your spelling/grammar.
- Have you cited all your references?
- Are all the references you have cited listed in full at the end of your essay?

Table 1.1 A guide to listing references

Type of reference	Example
From a book (one or two authors)	Surname(s) and initials, date of publication, title and edition of book, place of publication and publisher, e.g.
	Stude NT and Tuto R (2000) *Referencing For Fun* (2e). Cambridge University Press, Cambridge.
From a journal (one or two authors)	Surname(s) and initials, date of publication, title of article, journal name, volume and issue number (or date), pagination of article, e.g.
	Youcando IT (2001) Practice makes it easy. *Journal of Professional Studies* **5**(3): 23–27.
Three or more authors	Use the same formats shown above but instead of listing all the authors in the text cite the first three and then use *et al.* (Latin for 'and others'), e.g.
	(Smile, Grin, Laugh *et al.* 2002)
	whereas in the reference list:
	Smile Y, Grin M, Laugh J, Cry W, Weep N, Cheer H (2002) *Don't Worry, Be Happy*. American Press, New York.
From the internet	This is a new area; current practice is to provide author(s) surname(s) and initial(s), article title, website address (underscored) and the date it was accessed, e.g.
	Foster P and Jolley J. Report on wind farms. www.countryguardian.net accessed 05.08.02.

- Do your arguments follow on logically from each other?
- Ask a friend to read it, can they follow your arguments?
- Re-write your essay, or edit on your computer.
- Scream hysterically, run round the room, punching your fist in the air and shouting, '*Yes! I did it!*'

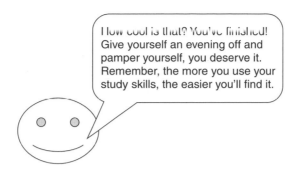

FINAL THOUGHTS

Hopefully after reading this chapter, you are confident that you can write a wonderful essay. However, there is just a vague chance that you might feel a bit overwhelmed by it all! *Don't worry! So will everyone else!* Expressing yourself in a formal way is a skill you need to learn and you will only learn by doing it. So *go for it!* Don't expect miracles to start with, but know that with practice it will become less scary until eventually academic writing will be second nature to you and you will not have to think about the process at all.

FURTHER READING

WEBSITES

- www.essaypunch.com This is an excellent site. It is interactive and set up to help you practise the essay writing process giving you tips along the way.
- www.write-an-essay.com A basic guide to essay writing but useful for the links it has to other sites, which are constantly expanding.

BOOKS

- Barrass R (2000) *Students Must Write* (2e) Routledge, London. This book looks at the topics covered above, but in more depth. It includes a guide to giving presentations and to answering essay questions under exam conditions. Clearly set out and readable.

REFERENCES

British Crime Survey www.homeoffice.gov.uk/rds/bcs1.html accessed on 05.08.02.
Hartley J (2001) New directions for study. *Psychology Review.* **8**: 20–21.
Holford P (1997) *The Optimum Nutrition Bible*. Piatkus, London.

Chapter 2

MANAGING YOUR OWN LEARNING

Gareth Owens

INTRODUCTION

This chapter looks at ways in which you can develop your own knowledge and practice to become more effective as a healthcare worker. It examines the process by which people learn and then helps you to relate this information to your particular learning style. The chapter emphasises that you learn best when you accept responsibility for your own development, and it offers a range of activities to help you to do this. The content relates to many of the knowledge and performance requirements of element two of the National Vocational Qualification (NVQ) unit CU7: 'Develop one's own values, priorities, interests and effectiveness'.

HOW PEOPLE LEARN

When considering how you may develop your practice more easily, it may be useful to consider learning as a process. Kolb (1984) described this process as a continuous cycle made up of four stages, as illustrated in Figure 2.1.

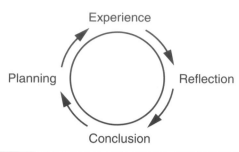

Experience	The first stage is to recall the actual experience you want to learn from.
Reflection	Next, consider all the relevant features of this experience: what went well; what didn't; how you felt about it, etc
Conclusion	Then, draw conclusions from the thoughts you made at the reflection stage. That is, identify the lessons you have learnt.
Planning	Plan to do something about your conclusions. Look to apply what you have learnt to your practice so that when the situation arises again you can deal with it more effectively.

Figure 2.1   The four stages of the learning cycle. (After Kolb, 1984.)

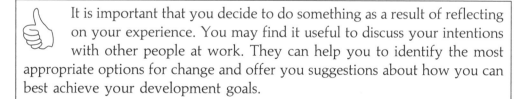

It is important that you decide to do something as a result of reflecting on your experience. You may find it useful to discuss your intentions with other people at work. They can help you to identify the most appropriate options for change and offer you suggestions about how you can best achieve your development goals.

USE OF A REFLECTION NOTE TO HELP YOU LEARN FROM EXPERIENCE

An important aspect of self-development is to be more aware of learning opportunities occurring and then to reflect on these in a systematic way. Keeping a record of your reflections is a useful way of making the most of the events that happen during your everyday practice. An example of such a reflection note is shown in Box 2.1. You can see that the four sections encourage you to move around the learning cycle, leading you from your experience at work to the planning for improvement stage.

Box 2.1   Example of a reflection note

Describe the experience   **Date:** . . . .

This morning, after two days on the ward, Mrs A died suddenly. A little while later, I spoke to her husband and asked him if there was going to be anyone to meet him when he got home. He reacted very angrily towards me, commenting that it was none of my business and that I needn't pretend that I cared anyway. Although I tried to reassure him that we were all concerned about him, he remained angry and asked me to leave the room.

I left and reported back to the nurse that Mr A had been distressed and unwilling to talk to me. I also mentioned that, from previous discussions with him, I had learnt that he had lived alone with his wife and that his family were a long way away.

Reflect on the experience (thoughts, feelings, behaviour)

At first, I felt hurt and upset that Mr A had spoken to me like that. For a short while I was also angry that I was shouted at when I was only trying to help and show him concern. But I also suspected that I had not fully understood the situation and had, somehow, 'put my foot in it'. Maybe, I had been naïve to expect that everyone would react to the death of a loved one in the same way. Looking back, I think I talked too much and maybe I should have let him get things off his chest, instead of trying to convince him I meant well. I did the right thing reporting my concerns about Mr A to the nurse. She helped me to understand that his reaction was a normal part of the grieving process and mentioned a book that explained this in more detail.

What did I learn/discover?
- That people react to loss differently and that anger is a normal part of the grieving process.
- That I have a tendency to take a patient's reaction or criticism too personally; I should try to recognise when they are expressing an understandable reaction to the situation in which they find themselves.
- The importance of giving time to listen to someone's concerns, rather than talking too much myself.
- That it is beneficial to talk through my experiences on the ward with another person.

What am I going to do about it?
- Learn more about people's reaction to loss by reading the chapter recommended by the nurse and by looking for further books in the library.
- Practise listening to patients more, so that I can begin to understand things from their point of view.
- Ask if there is anyone on the ward who I can go to whenever I need to discuss issues that come up at work.

Learning from experience

- Recall an incident that occurred at work during the last month. It may have been one that was particularly demanding or that caused you concern or, alternatively, it may have been something that went very well.
- Complete a reflection note for this incident.

When filling our the reflection note you may want to ask yourself questions similar to the following.

- Describe the experience:
    - What happened? Clarify the main features of the incident.
    - Why is this experience important to you?

- Reflect on what happened:
    - What went well and what didn't
    - Why did you act in the way you did?
    - How else could you have acted; what choices did you have?
    - How did you feel about the experience when it was happening?

- Conclusion:
    - What have you learnt from reflecting on this experience; what sense can you make of the situation?
    - How do you feel about the experience now?
    - What have you studied that might throw light on the situation?

- Plan:
    - What are you going to do about what you have learned?
    - If the same situation arose again what would you do?
    - Is there any further knowledge or skills that you need to develop?

(A blank reflection note for you to complete may be found at the end of this chapter; Appendix I.)

 If you are undertaking an NVQ, you may also want to use reflective notes as an evidence-gathering method. If so, they would be useful as a supplement to support other evidence or when observation of performance by the assessor is not appropriate.

THE SELF-COACHING CIRCLE

This self-development tool is also based upon the four stages of the learning cycle. It may be used not only to help you reflect upon a particular experience but also to identify how you could do things better next time. You may, therefore, find it useful when you need to solve a particular problem or improve your performance at work.

Figure 2.2 shows an example of a completed self-coaching circle form that has been adapted from Gillen (2000). A blank one may be found at the end of this chapter (*see* Appendix II). If you wish to try out this technique, the following notes will guide you through the process. When completing the form, just note a few points down rather than give a full description.

THE ISSUE OR TOPIC (BOX 1)

Here, identify the issue or topic you have chosen to explore. This should be a work-related activity that you often perform but would like to improve in some way. For example, 'completing work that is delegated to me on time'.

WHAT IS GOOD OR SUCCESSFUL PERFORMANCE? (BOX 2)

Briefly describe what would be seen as good performance, with regard to your chosen topic. That is, what would you be doing well?

WHAT WORKED WELL? (BOX 3)

Think back to the last time you performed this activity and write a list of things you did which resembled the descriptions in Box 2, or things about your actions with which you were pleased.

WHAT COULD HAVE WORKED BETTER? (BOX 4)

Again, think back to your previous performance, but this time note down what could have worked better or what you could have done differently?

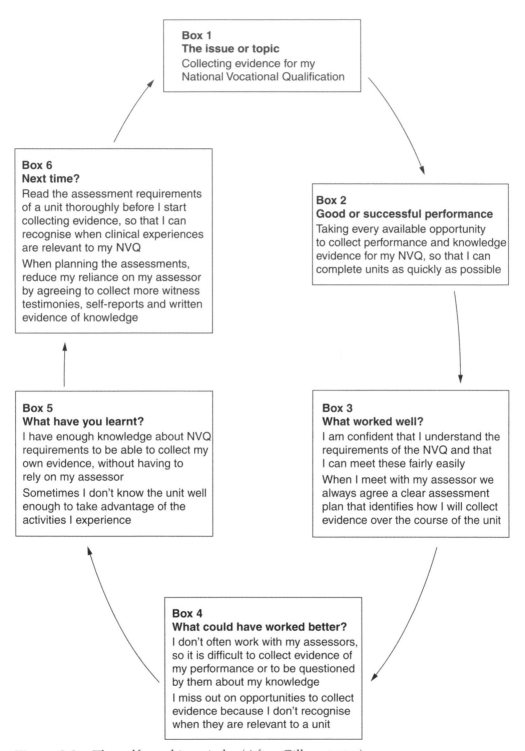

Figure 2.2 The self-coaching circle. (After Gillen, 2000.)

WHAT HAVE YOU LEARNT? (BOX 5)

Review what you have written so far and list what you have learnt.

NEXT TIME?

Lastly, make a few notes about what you will do to improve your performance in the future. Ask yourself: *'If I do what I have written in Box 6, will I do a better job next time?'*

LEARNING STYLES

People differ in the way they prefer to learn. For example, are you a 'hands on' style of learner who prefers to have a go and learn through trial and error, or would you rather find out as much as possible about something before deciding what to do next? Most of us probably use a mix of learning styles in different situations. But often, we rely heavily on one preferred learning style, because it is what we are most comfortable with. It is useful to be aware of your preferred learning style, because:

- you will then know what type of activity will make learning easier for you
- you will become aware of other learning activities that you are not using to their full advantage.

Honey and Mumford (1983) identified four main learning styles, which they based on Kolb's learning cycle. They called these styles 'Activist', 'Reflector', 'Theorist' and 'Pragmatist'.

ACTIVISTS

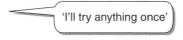

'I'll try anything once'

If you prefer this learning style, you like to learn by doing, and to work things out 'on the hoof'. You like to have a go, and tend to act first and consider the consequences later. You like to fill your days with activity and learn best when there is a lot of excitement and a range of changing things to tackle, usually involving people.

REFLECTORS

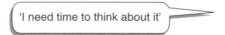

'I need time to think about it'

You like to absorb information and then think about it. You are likely to learn best from situations where you can stand back from events and listen and observe. You like to think before acting. Although you collect and analyse information about a subject thoroughly, you have a tendency to postpone reaching definitive conclusions for as long as possible.

THEORISTS

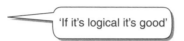

'If it's logical it's good'

You like interesting concepts, even if these are not immediately relevant. You like to draw conclusions from your observations and fit these into logical theories. You like activities to have a clear structure and purpose, and you like to question how things are done. You prefer logical, rational argument.

PRAGMATISTS

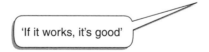

'If it works, it's good'

If you are a pragmatist, you are a person who likes to learn practical things and is interested in what works, what gives results. You are enthusiastic to try out ideas and see if they work out in practice. You tend to be impatient with extensive discussion and prefer to act quickly on ideas.

 Consider your preferred style of learning

The following checklist describes the four learning styles identified by Honey and Mumford (1983). To help find out what sort of learner you are:

- compare your behaviour and attitude at work with the statements listed below
- if you agree with a statement more than you disagree with it, put a tick in the appropriate box; if you disagree more that you agree, leave the box blank
- count up the ticks for each section and put the total in the appropriate box
- the section with the most ticks is your preferred learning style.

Activist	✓	Reflector	✓
I would describe myself as mostly: 'receptive, feeling, accepting, intuitive, present-orientated'	☐	I would describe myself as mostly 'tentative, watching, observing, reflecting, reserved'	☐
I'll try anything once	☐	I need time to 'think about it'	☐
I enjoy challenges and can work quickly	☐	I pay a great attention to detail in all I do.	☐
I get bored easily and enjoy moving on to new things	☐	I can spend a lot of time thinking about work without actually getting down to it	☐
I am comfortable working without timetables or plans	☐	I am careful not to jump to conclusions too quickly	☐
I learn by talking ideas through with other people	☐	I think that decisions made on a thorough analysis of all the information are sounder than those based on intuition	☐
I prefer to skip-read; trying to absorb everything is a waste of time	☐	If I have to write something I would tend to produce lots of reports before settling on a final one	☐
I prefer to respond to events in a spontaneous, flexible way rather than to plan things in advance	☐	Its best to think carefully before taking an action	☐
Total		**Total**	

Theorist	✓	Pragmatist	✓
I would describe myself as mostly: 'analytical, thinking, logical, rational'	☐	I would describe myself as mostly: 'practical, doing, active, responsible'	☐
If it's logical it's good	☐	If it works, it's good	☐
I tend to be uncomfortable unless things are tidy and fit into a rational scheme	☐	I look for a link between the subject matter and a real problem or opportunity at work	☐
I like to understand how things work and how ideas have been developed	☐	I like to 'see results'	☐

I like reading for ideas ☐	When I hear about a new idea or approach, I immediately start working out how to apply it in practice ☐
I enjoy making connections between different topics and finding out how ideas link together ☐	I can often see better, more practical ways to get things done ☐
I get on best with logical, analytical people and less well with spontaneous, 'irrational' people ☐	In discussions I like to get straight to the point ☐
In discussions with people I often find I am the most dispassionate and objective ☐	I don't mind hurting people's feelings so long as the job gets done ☐
Total	**Total**

There is no best style of learning – each has its advantages and disadvantages. However, if you know your style, you can build upon your strengths and work towards improving the areas that are not developed.

 Developing your learning style

Identify your preferred learning style(s) at the top of the blank form 'Developing your learning style' (Appendix III):

- in the top left-hand box, write out the strengths or advantages of having this learning style
- in the top right-hand box, identify its weaknesses and disadvantages
- in the bottom box think about how you can broaden your learning style to include the learning styles on which you scored less highly.

If you want to find out more about learning styles visit the website www.peterhoneylearning.com where you will find more comprehensive questionnaires to complete.

FINAL THOUGHTS

In busy clinical areas, it is not always possible to be released to attend study days. But there are sufficient opportunities for development within the workplace –

If you accept responsibility for your own development. This chapter has introduced several ideas and techniques that will help you make the most of your day-to-day experiences, so that you may continue to improve your knowledge and skills without having to rely on others for support.

REFERENCES

Gillen T (2000) *The Coaching Skills Activity Pack*. Fenman Ltd, Ely.

Honey P and Mumford A (1983) *Using Your Learning Styles*. Peter Honey Publications, Maidenhead.

Kolb D (1984) *Experiential Learning: Experience as the source of learning and development*. Prentice-Hall, Englewood Cliffs, NJ.

APPENDIX I

REFLECTION NOTE

Describe the experience	**Date:** . . . . . .

Reflect on the experience (thoughts, feelings, behaviour)

What did I learn/discover?

What am I going to do about it?

APPENDIX II

THE SELF-COACHING CIRCLE

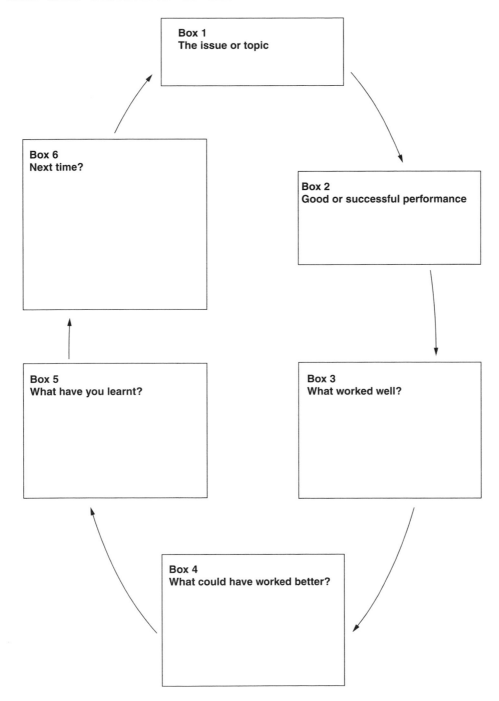

Box 1
The issue or topic

Box 6
Next time?

Box 2
Good or successful performance

Box 5
What have you learnt?

Box 3
What worked well?

Box 4
What could have worked better?

APPENDIX III

DEVELOPING YOUR LEARNING STYLE

My preferred learning style: . . . .

Strengths/advantages	Weaknesses/disadvantages
How can my learning style be broadened?	

Chapter 3

COMMUNICATION

Claire Evans and Sam Donohue

INTRODUCTION

A broad definition of communication is 'the giving and receiving of information'. Historically, patients have often had little say in their care. In modern healthcare the goal is patients being partners in their care, making informed choices and feeling valued, respected and empowered.

This chapter concentrates on how we give and receive information and how this enables us to interact effectively with others. Throughout this chapter activities have been developed to equip you with the necessary skills to communicate effectively within your healthcare environment.

WHY IS COMMUNICATION IMPORTANT?

Communication needs to be effective for patients to feel listened to. Communication is not just limited to our patients and colleagues but also extends to patients' relatives and friends.

Complaints are sometimes made and, in general, the reason for them is a breakdown in communication, such as lack of information or staff appearing not to listen or not appearing concerned about a situation.

For communication to be effective the relationship between healthcare professionals and patients needs certain ground rules. Figure 3.1 identifies some of these.

In effective relationships people feel:

- valued
- informed

- empowered
- respected
- partners in their care.

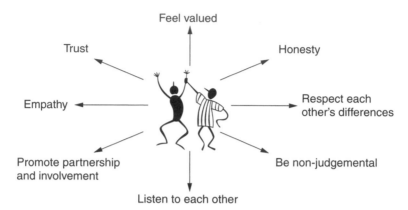

Figure 3.1 Some ground rules for effective communication between healthcare professionals and patients.

Healthcare professionals should be:

- non-judgemental
- respectful of others and their differences
- self-aware
- able to empower others
- honest and flexible.

WHEN DOES THE PROCESS OF COMMUNICATION BEGIN?

In order to understand our development and needs as human beings we should look at, and be more aware of, the start of the communication process. As carers we often experience situations where individuals may not be able to communicate easily or effectively and we may need to adapt our communication skills as necessary.

FORMS OF COMMUNICATION

There are various forms of communication:

- verbal – voice/tone/volume
- non-verbal (body language)

- telephone
- information technology (IT)
- written documentation.

VERBAL AND NON-VERBAL COMMUNICATIONS

The process of communication is littered with subtle non-verbal messages that influence the meaning of interaction. Verbal communication, that is, expressing ourselves by tone and pitch of the voice, and non-verbal communication, expressing ourselves by eye contact, facial expressions, gestures, tone of voice, proximity and physical touch. From non-verbal communication we can express our thoughts and feelings.

TELEPHONE

For some people the telephone is their primary link to the outside world; they may not be able to visit their relatives because of their own ill health or the distance they would have to travel. When they phone your clinical area they will have certain expectations of you and the information they are about to receive. For example, they will expect to feel welcome and not a nuisance, and to gain an adequate amount of information and feel satisfied. Remember, when you talk on the telephone the only communication medium available is your voice – this means that the listener will elicit information from the tone, pitch and pace of your voice.

 Obtaining information

If you telephoned a hospital ward to try to find out information about your relative, what would your expectations be? Write them down.

 Remember the following when you speak to someone on the telephone.

- Be prepared when answering the telephone:
  - finish your conversation if you are talking to someone
  - have a piece of paper and pen ready for messages
  - know how to use the telephone and how to transfer calls.

- Introduction:
  - introduce yourself and the area where you are (for example the ward or department)
  - give an opening and welcoming statement.
- Give an informed answer – if you do not know the information, find out and try to be as co-operative as possible.
- Maintain confidentiality and if necessary take the caller's number to return their call and give the required information to prevent them from waiting on the line.
- Thank the caller for their enquiry and assistance.

 If a patient has a large network of friends and family telephoning you could suggest that they nominate one member to call on their behalf to obtain an update in information, or that they take it in turns to call. You could also suggest when it would be a good time to call during the day.

INFORMATION TECHNOLOGY (IT)

This is a very useful and powerful source of communication and information. More and more patients are now turning to the internet for information. For example, NHS Direct has been expanded to include a major internet site that provides online advice and health promotion information. It is designed to relieve some of the pressures on acute hospitals and primary care teams.

Another example of IT communication is the launch of hand-held computers and electronic patient records for healthcare professionals to share documentation and to communicate and practise more effectively ('seamless care').

WRITTEN DOCUMENTATION

Documentation and report writing are central to communication and the continuity of care. Unfortunately, notes are not always up to date or they do not contain adequate information. Castledine (1998) states that documentation 'is a method of assembling records to authenticate what we have done and the reasons behind our actions'. Healthcare professionals have a professional duty to produce good-quality and accurate documentation. The Nursing and Midwifery Council (NMC) has produced a booklet, *Guidelines for Records and Record Keeping 2002* (NMC, 2001), that outlines what should be included in documentation and the standard required, and which states that records must be:

- accurate
- written as one is caring for the patient and following the care given
- accurately timed, dated and signed
- free from correction fluid, and if an error is made, a single line to be drawn through the incorrect writing
- clearly written in a manner that cannot be erased
- free from jargon and abbreviations
- free from offensive subjective statements
- legible for patients.

Records should also identify problems that have arisen and the action taken to rectify them.

It is worth noting that, in some clinical settings, healthcare professionals are expected to write patients' care plans and evaluation notes. Generally, if this is the accepted standard a registered member of staff should always countersign notes and care plans.

GIVING, RECEIVING AND RETRIEVING INFORMATION

When information is to be provided, many factors should be considered:

- when the information is to be provided, and how often
- where the information is to be given and within what environment
- in what form – verbal, leaflets, CD ROM or video
- over what period of time (considering a person's attention span)
- the language used – free from jargon, clear and concise
- level of understanding of the person – should be checked before, during and after providing the information
- the individual's needs – will an interpreter be required or any special aids, such as picture boards or computers?
- any other supporting information to back up key points.

Table 3.1 How our senses affect memory

We remember:
25% of what we hear
30% of what we see
50% of what we see and hear
80% of what we see, hear and do or experience

As individuals we learn in many different ways. Our ability to remember things is also variable depending on how the information was originally taken in. Table 3.1 identifies how our senses affect memory.

TOOLS FOR GIVING, RECEIVING AND RETRIEVING INFORMATION

QUESTIONS

Asking questions is particularly important in healthcare because it is the only way we can obtain information from, and increase our understanding of, patients' healthcare needs.

Open questions
Open questions are used to elicit information from patients and cannot normally be answered by a 'yes' or 'no' answer. The answers are normally longer and unpredictable. Open questions allow clients to express themselves and encourage them to discuss their feelings and thoughts. They start with the words *What* or *How*, for example, '*How do you feel about your treatment?*' or '*What do you think about that information?*'.

Closed questions
These questions usually obtain a one-word answer, either 'yes' or 'no'. They are used for obtaining specific information and are quite predictable. They are helpful if patients have limited understanding or are unable to express themselves because of communication difficulties or extreme pain. Closed questions include, '*What is your name?*' or '*Are you in pain?*'.

Listening
Listening is perhaps the most important of all skills when working with people. In order to build effective relationships with your patients there are certain responses you can use whilst listening.

Summarising and reflecting back
Repeating back what has been said to you by patients and what you think they mean. This clarifies patients' main points and prevents any misunderstandings.

Appropriate silences
This allows patients time to think what they want to say and to express themselves. This can be quite uncomfortable at first but it takes pressure away from patients and is really beneficial.

Body language
This can be crucial when patients are trying to confide in you or you are trying to obtain information from them. Body language can show empathy, interest and concern. A good posture for active listening is nodding encouragingly, sitting near to patients and facing them to one side.

BODY LANGUAGE

Your body language is a very powerful form of non-verbal communication that relays messages about how you are thinking and feeling.
Forms of body language include:

- facial expression – happy, sad, angry, puzzled or confused
- hand gestures (such as 'thumbs up')
- posture – facing away or arms crossed in a defensive action
- movements – shrugging shoulders, fidgeting or pacing up and down
- eye contact.

What messages do we convey through our body language?

- boredom
- anxiety
- agitation
- pleasure
- confusion
- sadness
- pain.

 Communicating

- Can you think of any other ways of communicating?
- Are you aware of any particular ways you express your feelings through your body language?

ZONES OF INTERACTION

Zones are found around our body and form the acceptable boundaries between ourselves and those with whom we are communicating. The zones consist of the following (Figure 3.2).

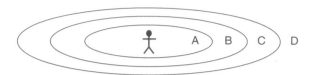

Figure 3.2   Zones of interaction.

- *Intimate zone* (A) – up to 46 cm (18 inches) from the body. To enter this space one would have to gain patients' trust otherwise intrusion may cause embarrassment or discomfort.
- *Personal zone* (B) – between 46–124 cm (18 inches and 4 feet). This zone is sometimes referred to as 'personal space' and boundaries may move, depending on the setting and situation.
- *Social zone* (C) – found between 124–372 cm (4 and 12 feet). This may be experienced in a meeting or conversational setting where touch would not be possible; it may be a more formal occasion.
- *Public zone* (D) – this space may extend from 372 cm (12 feet). Experienced at meetings and gatherings.

You can see from the different zones how different messages may be conveyed. If you were interested in a patient and wanted to engage in conversation you would approach, if appropriate, into their personal zone. However, if you stood within their social or public zone it could appear you were being very formal and unwilling to participate in conversation. Be aware, however, that patients can feel very vulnerable and uncomfortable in a clinical setting for a number of reasons so may feel sensitive to people approaching into the intimate or personal zone.

  Effective communication

Mabel is normally a cheerful and chatty lady but today appears quiet and withdrawn. The nurse looking after Mabel approached the end of her bed and asked her if she was alright whilst looking at Mabel's drug chart. Mabel replied she was fine and looked away. The nurse seemed happy with this and said she would see her later and moved on to the next patient.

How do you think this situation was handled and could it have been dealt with more effectively?

Consider the following points.

- What is Mabel's body language communicating to you? Is Mabel showing signs of pain or discomfort? What are her facial expressions?
- How would you approach Mabel?
- Where would you sit, and in what way?
- Tone of voice – what does it tell you about Mabel's mood and how can you be reassuring and comforting to Mabel through your tone of voice?
- How can you demonstrate your interest in Mabel and that you are listening to her?

 Recognise the lack of sensory stimuli that patients can experience, which can lead to boredom and becoming withdrawn. Assess your clinical environment. It is conducive to effective communication or could it be improved?

BARRIERS TO COMMUNICATION IN HEALTHCARE

Barriers can prevent effective communication. Commonly, these are referred to as 'internal' and 'external' barriers. Internal barriers stem from within individuals; external barriers originate outside individuals, examples of these may be seen in Table 3.2.

Table 3.2 Barriers to communication

Internal	External
Prejudice	Noise (telephone, people talking, music or television in the background)
Assumptions	Environmental (lack of privacy, inappropriate area, extremes in temperature)
Transference	Language (accents, colloquialisms)
Labelling	Distractions
Judging	Interruptions
Having your own agenda	

Barriers to communication

Think about your own clinical area. What barriers are there to communicating effectively? Can you think of any solutions to overcome these barriers?

How would you discuss your thoughts and findings with other members of your team?

ADAPTING COMMUNICATION SKILLS

There are times when you may need to adapt your communication style to the needs of individuals. These may include communicating with someone who has:

- hearing impairment
- visual impairment
- dysphasia (*see* p. 40)
- aphasia (*see* p. 40)
- learning difficulties
- language difficulties
- gender differences.

 Prepare the environment the best you can to aid effective communication. Assess the best form of communication according to the needs of the patient and the environment. Also, document all care and communication skills to promote continuity and tailoring care to the needs of the individual.

PROMOTING EFFECTIVE COMMUNICATION

Remember your communication skills:

- maintain eye contact
- open and receptive body language and positioning

- reduce distractions
- utilise other forms of communication
- use an interpreter or sign language
- gestures.

AIDS TO COMMUNICATION

Aids can enhance your communication and help the other person understand and retain information. They can also help them communicate with you and express their needs and wishes. Examples of aids are:

- written material (such as leaflets)
- picture boards
- illustrated menus
- system of gestures
- word book of everyday activities
- pen and paper
- interpreters
- glasses, hearing aids
- showing items to assist information-sharing
- videophone to provide a remote real-time interpreting service via a computer fitted with a digital camera.

You may also use other members from the team as a resource and for reference, for example speech and language therapists or occupational therapists.

To help you to understand some of the issues identified earlier in this chapter you may find the following information useful.

Hearing impairment

In the UK there are 8.7 million people with hearing loss – that is one in seven (Mangan and Robins, 1999). Many use hearing aids and lip-read to aid communication. As many as 70 000 people use British Sign Language (BSL). If you are communicating with a person who has a hearing impairment then remember the following.

- *Positioning* – face the light, on the same level as the person so that they can see your facial expressions and lips when talking.
- *Talk slowly* – but do not shout as this can distort speech.

- *Maintain eye contact* – at all times to check understanding and to show interest.
- Reduce distractions.
- *Hearing aid* – if one is worn ensure this is maintained with a battery and check that it is fitted into the correct ear. You can then talk at the correct side of the patient.
- *Be aware* – some patients may hide their disability because they are self-conscious.
- *Provide written material* – to back up your points.
- *Use gestures* – to reinforce the information.
- *Be aware* – some patients may have real difficulty in understanding staff with strong accents.

Visual impairment

Although the overall incidence of visual impairment in the UK is unknown, the Royal College of Ophthalmologists reports that there is an increase in the occurrence of cataracts, glaucoma and degeneration of the retina in people aged over 65 years. It is thought that the numbers registering for blindness and partial sight represent less than 50% of the real extent of the problem (Office of Population Censuses and Surveys, 1999). Again, if you are communicating with a person who has a visual impairment, remember the following.

- *Use touch* – to let the client know you have approached and to attract their attention.
- *Identify* – and introduce yourself.
- *Explain* – all your actions.
- *Provide information* – in the form of Braille or tape to listen to.
- *Consider* – room sizes, acoustics, furniture layout and décor.
- *Extra help* – do they have a friend or relative who can hand sign?

Dysphasia or aphasia

Nearly 75% of all strokes occur in people aged 65 years or over, and nearly 60% of those who survive a stroke experience speech and language difficulties (Kopp, 2001). Reading and writing may also be affected, as may facial expression and control over tone and emphasis of the voice. Dysphasia is a language impairment – affecting people's ability to express themselves and to understand another's language. At times it can be severe enough not to be able to make themselves understood at all. So:

- take time talking to clients and repeat if necessary
- be patient

- use communication aids
- reduce the amount of distractions around if possible
- adapt your questioning style, for example use closed questions.

Language differences
When communicating with people whose first language is different:

- use an interpreter
- ask if the family can provide a list of key words to refer to
- provide written material in the form of books or leaflets
- be aware of the different use of gestures in other cultures
- do not make assumptions about patients' wishes or understanding because of their culture or appearance, discuss patients' needs and wishes with them.

Lastly, take care to ensure that patients' views *are* being put forward by those acting as interpreters and that any decision taken *does* involve patients' views.

Learning difficulties
Again, remember to:

- use simple words and short sentences
- repeat if necessary
- involve family and carers to promote continuity
- build and gain trust.

GENDER DIFFERENCES

Be aware of the differences between genders and the way individuals express themselves, but again, do not make assumptions.

FINAL THOUGHTS

Communication is one of the most important caring skills as it allows us to improve our understanding of patients' needs. Remember, we are in partnership with our patients and, by involving patients directly in their care through good communication and information, patients are able to be part of the decision-making process.

REFERENCES

Castledine G (1995) *Writing, Documentation and Communication for Nurses*. Quay Books, Swindon.

Kopp P (2001) Better communication with older patients. *Professional Nurse*. **16**(8): 1296–99.

Mangan M and Robins J (1999) Seen and not heard. *Nursing Times*. **95**(37): 10–12.

Nursing and Midwifery Council (2001) *Guidelines for Record and Record Keeping (2002)*. NMC, London.

Office of Population Census and Surveys (1999) The prevalence of disability among adults. In: *Surveys of Disability in Great Britain*. The Stationery Office, London.

Chapter 4

PROMOTING THE EQUALITY, DIVERSITY AND RIGHTS OF PEOPLE IN HEALTHCARE

Sam Donohue and Claire Evans

INTRODUCTION

If you took your car into the local garage for a service you expect to be treated the same whether you have an old banger or the latest model. Similarly, if you arrive at a restaurant you expect to be greeted and treated the same, no matter what you look like, sound like or whom you are with.

When individuals enter a healthcare environment these expectations continue. When you arrive at your doctor's surgery you expect to be treated courteously, to have choices and to receive care that is equal to that offered to the other clients, regardless of your culture, gender, physical or mental ability and socio-economic status.

This chapter focuses on the role of support workers in promoting the rights of individuals in healthcare. Issues such as discrimination and prejudice, as well as advocacy, consent, confidentiality and making a complaint, are all explored here.

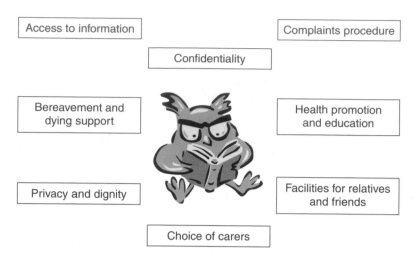

Figure 4.1   Human rights in healthcare.

HUMAN RIGHTS

'Human rights' may be defined as rights to which we are all *equally* entitled. In 1988 the Human Rights Act was passed; it came into force in October 2000. This was seen as a milestone as it meant that certain rights could be enforced legally and any breach may be brought to the courts.

Human rights include:

- the right to life (article 2)
- the prohibition of torture and inhuman and degrading treatment (article 3)
- the right to liberty (article 5)
- the right to respect for privacy and family life (article 8)
- freedom of expression (article 10)
- the prohibition of discrimination (article 14).

Figure 4.1 illustrates each client's equal rights in healthcare.

 The rights people have when entering a healthcare environment are clearly laid out, but what about their expectations? They may also be entitled to expect certain standards, such as a hygienic environment and courteous staff.

Expectations
Can you think of any other expectations people have when they enter a healthcare environment? List them.

PREJUDICE AND DISCRIMINATION

Throughout our lives we may experience prejudice, discrimination, isolation or harassment. This may occur at school, in the workplace or socially, in fact, in a variety of everyday environments. In healthcare we expect to be treated equally. To understand how we can promote equal treatment we first need to understand the key concepts of prejudice and discrimination and how they exist in society, as well as the responsibilities of individuals and organisations when ensuring that all individuals are treated equally within healthcare.

Prejudice may be defined as a view about others that has been developed from pre-conceived ideas, societal stereotypes, ignorance and misunderstanding.

Prejudices can inform discrimination. By this we mean that individuals may discriminate – choose between alternatives – on the basis of prejudices that they have developed.

Discrimination may be categorised as direct or indirect.

Direct discrimination occurs when people are treated less favourably on the grounds of sex, race, ethnicity, disability or sexual orientation. To discriminate against a person on grounds of sex, race or disability is UNLAWFUL.

Indirect discrimination is found when unnecessary particulars are insisted upon that, in turn, will discriminate against a particular group of people.

Discrimination may also be used positively or negatively. *Positive* discrimination involves asking for a particular individual in response to the needs of a particular group. The 'genuine occupational qualification' allows an employer to discriminate if the post requires it. For example, you may see an advert for a diabetic specialist nurse who speaks Urdu – this may be in response to the needs of the local population. The education of the population and prevention of diabetes would be hindered if the applicant could not speak the predominant language of the client group. Other examples are found occasionally, for example an employer can state a particular sex for a position, if the post-holder will work in a single-sex establishment or if the post requires activities which can be provided more effectively by one sex. *Negative* discrimination may be seen in society at an individual level, where one individual treats another differently because of their lifestyle or external characteristics. It also exists at a broader societal level, where long-established systems have a negative effect on equality.

Examples of legislation to promote anti-discriminatory practice

Race Relations (Amendment) Act 2000
Human Rights Act 1998
Trade Union and Employees Rights Act 1993

The Criminal Justice Act 1992
The National Health Service and Community Care Act 1990
The Children Act 1989
The Employment Act 1988
The Disabled Person's Act 1986
The Mental Health Act 1983
Education (Handicapped Children) Act 1980
The Race Relations Act 1976
The Equal Pay Act 1975
The Sex Discrimination Act 1975
The Sexual Offences Act 1967
The Local Government Act 1966

 Discrimination

Can you think of a time when you have witnessed or experienced prejudice or discrimination?

How did you feel?

What did you do?

In order to protect individuals entering a healthcare environment each organisation has certain responsibilities that they expect themselves and their employees to abide by.

Organisations must:

- ensure that all individuals have equal opportunities, irrespective of age, gender, nationality, religion, sexual orientation, colour or disability

- ensure that all employees have equal opportunities in terms of recruitment, selection, training, promotion, appraisal, work allocation and career management.

Individuals must:

- be responsible for their own behaviour
- be aware of their own attitudes and how they can affect their judgement
- not harass, bully, abuse or victimise anyone
- challenge any discriminatory or offensive remarks.

 Responsibilities

A patient says to you that he does not want 'that foreign doctor' looking after him.

What are your responsibilities to the patient and to the doctor?

What are the organisational responsibilities to the patient and to the doctor?

Remember, if you witness discrimination but do not act to stop it then you are as culpable as the person who is acting in a discriminatory way. Patients are entitled to choices concerning who looks after them. However, these choices cannot be based on prejudice. Try to find out why a patient does not want a particular doctor looking after them. If there is a valid reason then this should be addressed, if not then the organisation has a duty to protect the doctor from discrimination and prejudice.

So, what happens when individuals receiving healthcare cannot protect their own rights? As healthcare professionals we should always ensure that we act in the best interest of patients or clients; however, there may be times when a person needs some help to express their needs and wishes and in this situation a patient may use an *advocate*.

ADVOCACY

Advocacy literally means 'to call' (*ad* – to, *vocare* – call); 'an individual calls another to speak on their behalf'. The role of the advocate may be that of a go-between. An advocate may be used to express wishes or even to influence others on behalf of an individual (Figure 4.2). Bennett (1999) stresses that advocacy represents 'an expressed need by the patient, not a perceived need by the nurse'.* This means we cannot assume we are advocates or assume we know what patients wish.

 Advocacy

Have you ever acted as an advocate?
Why did someone ask you to speak on their behalf?
Did you feel the person benefited from your actions?

There are many situations in healthcare when individuals may need an advocate. For example, someone with mental health problems, a person with a learning disability, a child, a person who has problems communicating whether due to language or physical disability. However, we cannot generalise. Every individual must be treated equally, we must not assume that patients do or do not need an advocate. For example, an elderly lady says that she does not want

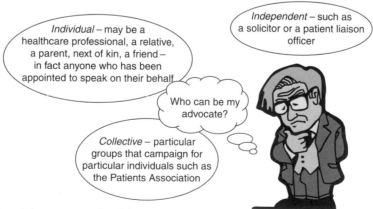

Figure 4.2   Advocates in healthcare.

*Bennett O (1999) Advocacy in nursing. *Nursing Standard*. **14**(11): 40–41.

to go home, she feels she can no longer cope. This may be the case but unpick what she is saying – is there anything else we can take from this scenario?

Before you make any assumptions and decide to speak on this lady's behalf find out the answers to the following questions.

- What else may she be feeling?
- Has she said this to anyone else? How would you find this out?
- Is she scared of being alone or does she not know what help is available?
- Does she truly wish to leave her home and live in residential care or does she feel that she is being a burden?

It may be that the conclusion to this scenario is that the lady does not want to go home and so she is discharged to a place of her choosing or it may be that with appropriate support, continuity of care, accurate documentation of her needs and wishes, and with input from all relevant members of the multi-disciplinary team she does return home. Either way her needs and wishes are followed and where necessary they are expressed by a person she feels suitable to be her advocate.

- Never assume that you are the best person to act as someone's advocate.
- Always document any wishes expressed by a person or any concerns that they have.
- Wherever possible offer continuity of care. If a person grows to know and trust you they are more likely to feel that their needs and wishes will be supported.

Remember, it is not your role to approve of the decision the patient is making, but to support the decision.

An example of a situation in which someone may need an advocate may be found when they are asked to give consent to a particular treatment, procedure or intervention.

CONSENT

Every person has a choice whether they have an investigation or examination. Healthcare professionals have a responsibility to provide sufficient, detailed information in a format that may be understood by the person to whom it is being presented. This is because *consent* is more than permission; it should be informed so that people can weigh up information and make choices that are right for them.

Consent may be divided into two forms:

- *Express consent* – verbal or written and is needed by law for surgical and invasive procedures.
- *Implied consent* – the form of consent with which you are most likely to be involved. A person will often imply consent for routine and non-invasive procedures. Yet even though consent is implied people still have choices.

  Express and implied consent

From assisting a person with their hygiene needs to testing their urine for infection, think of times where you assume consent or it is implied.

So, what can people expect when they are consenting to a procedure or treatment? Figure 4.3 makes some suggestions.

Remember, we need to be flexible, non-judgemental and aware of individual differences, which may be due to age, culture or religious beliefs. People are often consenting to life-changing procedures when they feel vulnerable and scared. Equally, they may be consenting to having their hair washed or their pressure areas checked – they still have choices and can expect that these be respected.

But what happens if a person cannot consent? To give legal consent you must:

- be over 18 years of age
- have received information concerning the procedure *and understood it*
- be giving consent voluntarily.

However, there are exceptions to the rules.

In an emergency the medical team is allowed to perform whatever procedure is needed to save a life but no more than that. However, if there is any prior knowledge that a person has particular wishes then these are legally binding. An example of this may be a person who is known to be a Jehovah's Witness and who needs a blood transfusion or a person that has clearly stated they do not wish to be resuscitated, in both of these cases in an emergency the medical team cannot decide to give the blood transfusion or to resuscitate.

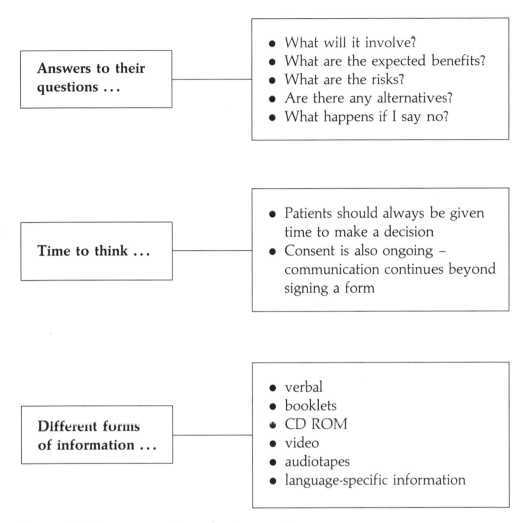

Figure 4.3 Some suggestions about consent.

Patient choice. The patient may choose not to hear all of the information concerning a procedure.

Mental incapacity. If a person is not able to make an informed decision owing to some form of mental incapacity then the law sees that they need to be protected. This may take the form of an advocate, such as a legal guardian or appointed next of kin. However, no one can give or withhold consent on behalf of a mentally incapacitated individual.

Age. A person under the age of 18 can consent to a procedure if they are seen to be 'mature'. This is normally defined by a court.

There are many grey areas when we consider consent and it is recommended that you visit the websites listed in Further Reading at the end of this chapter and read some of the referenced material.

The main role for the healthcare team is to ensure that people are treated as individuals, that they are given plenty of information and that they feel that their choices are valued. If you feel that someone has not consented then you should speak to your colleagues about it. Once they have expressed their wishes then make sure these are properly documented.

CONFIDENTIALITY

Another basic right we have when entering a healthcare setting is to be treated in a confidential manner. Imagine standing in a lift in a hospital, you are about to visit your father when you hear two doctors discussing him, his condition and his potential treatments. Or how about waiting in the health centre reception to overhear the practice nurse speaking to the hospital about your results. Now imagine you have just overheard midwives discussing your decision not to breastfeed your baby.

All these scenarios would anger us because we expect to have our personal information to be stored and disclosed in a confidential manner. Confidentiality in healthcare is crucial. It has an important role to play in:

- promoting trust and respect
- preserving dignity and self-esteem
- preventing exploitation.

It also ensures that when information is disclosed and shared it is done so in a recognised manner. Both clients and professionals understand what may and may not be disclosed and when this can or cannot occur. If any of the above scenarios occurred, our right to complain would be upheld.

We may also expect information to be stored securely, for it to be accurate, for it to be relevant and for it to be stored for as long as it is necessary and no longer.

Relevant legislation
Access to Personal Files Act 1987
Access to Medical Reports Act 1988
Public Interest Disclosure Act 1999
Data Protection Act 1998 (implemented 2000)

Confidentiality

Where is client information discussed in your area?

Is this area private?

Where is client information documented?

Does anyone have access to this information?

How could this be improved?

There are times when confidential information may need to be disclosed. This may usually be done with the agreement of the client, for example if the next of kin needs to know information but cannot attend the hospital or surgery. However, there are times when disclosure without the consent of the client may be allowed legally. Examples of this are disclosing information to the police under the Road Traffic Act 1988, disclosure in the public interest and disclosure before trial.

- Do not discuss clients or their care within earshot of others.
- Ensure all written documentation is stored securely.
- Ensure that any written documentation that is kept with the patient does not hold any confidential information.

- Be aware of the dangers of the telephone. If you must discuss confidential matters on the telephone then ensure:
  - the telephone is in a private environment
  - the client has consented to the information being given to that particular person
  - if possible phone them back to ensure you are speaking to the right person
  - only disclose the necessary information
  - urge the person to arrange to come to you or if not for you to go to them.

So what happens when things go wrong? There may be times when people do not feel that they have been treated fairly or equally.

MAKING A COMPLAINT

There are a number of factors that will cause individuals to complain, sometimes we encounter people who have different expectations and different standards. Patients should be seen as consumers of healthcare, they have rights and choices and these include being listened to and having action taken if things go wrong.

People complain for a number of reasons, but the following are seen most often:

- excessive waiting
- lack of information
- negligence or trespass
- conflict of information
- unexpected death or discharge
- loss of property or damage to property
- rudeness and arrogance of staff.

 Complaints

Can you think of two reasons why people have complained in your workplace?

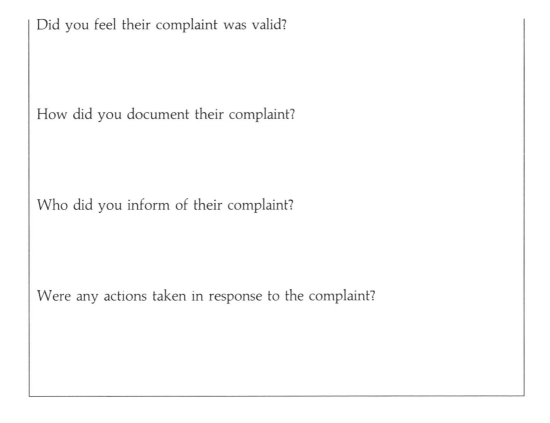

Did you feel their complaint was valid?

How did you document their complaint?

Who did you inform of their complaint?

Were any actions taken in response to the complaint?

There are many times when people feel dissatisfied and make a verbal complaint. So how can you stop a complaint escalating?

- Firstly, remember that complainants should be treated courteously and with respect.
- Try to use a quiet space and listen actively to what is being said.
- Try to isolate the problem and identify what the complainant is seeking.
- You may need to ask for a more senior member of staff to be involved.
- Ensure that you document what the complainant has said, what has been said by you and what further actions have been taken.

Whatever your feelings you must ensure that complainants have proper access to a complaints procedure – remember, do not take this personally – if you were in their shoes would you complain?

Your response will often be key in diffusing the situation. If the complaint needs to continue then the organisation has responsibilities. These include ensuring that a complaint is acknowledged within two days of receipt, that it is investigated and that learning occurs, that is, practice is changed if necessary.

Managing complaints

Bill has been waiting in the Outpatient Department for two hours. He was told to come in because his prostate symptoms were worsening. His wife is anxious and Bill is in pain. Whenever anyone in uniform walks past they do not look at them and Bill's wife is beginning to feel like they are invisible. She has asked a number of times what time they will be seen, but each person has given them different information. Bill's wife approaches the desk again where three staff are chatting; she appears angry and aggressive. She demands to see the manager of the department stating that it is a disgrace how they have been treated.

- What could the staff have done to avoid this happening?
- What actions need to be taken now?
- How can you calm Bill's wife down?
- What image of the department will she have when she leaves?

Now imagine you are Bill's wife, how would you feel? Add in the fact that Bill has diabetes and had not eaten for four hours, he was also told by the doctor that if his symptoms worsen it may mean that the cancer has returned and their daughter has just been admitted to hospital for investigations into respiratory problems.

Your role is to ensure that Bill and his wife are informed of what is happening. Do not walk past them without checking if they are OK and remember that what you are seeing may not be the full picture.

This was the worst scenario, as Bill's wife should have felt supported by the outpatient staff and not been forced into making a complaint and acting out of character.

Let us be realistic; there are times when we are frantic and have too many demands on our time.

- Explain what is happening – if you are busy, say so – warn people.
- Remember your basic communication skills – always be courteous, use open body language, smile and introduce yourself.

- Be sensitive and non-judgemental.
- Involve others if need be – a more senior member of staff or the Patient Advisory Liaison Service (PALS).
- Document everything.
- Do not take it personally but make sure you find out why a complaint is being made and learn from it.

Occasionally, people may not be in the position to complain. If they are patients our role is to protect them from ill treatment, if it is a member of staff our role is to encourage them to speak up – if not speak for them.

REPORTING BAD PRACTICE

We have all heard the horror stories of healthcare settings that were investigated because of reports of patient abuse. This chapter explores the rights of people entering a healthcare environment. However, what if you have worked with someone or are working with someone who does not appear to promote these rights?

It is your responsibility and duty to your patients to ensure that they are always treated equally and with respect, that they are given choices and have their human rights upheld.

This responsibility extends to intervening if these rights are not respected. If you ignore mistreatment or witness poor practice and fail to intervene then *you* are as culpable as the person committing the abuse. That means that you are also guilty of malpractice.

What constitutes mistreatment?

- *Denying basic rights* – such as food, fluid, meeting hygiene needs, a safe environment, medication or treatment.
- Routine restraint.
- *Discrimination* – including words used to refer to someone, facilities and treatment offered, and time spent with a person.
- Physical, sexual and verbal abuse.

So, what should you do?

- *Report it to your manager* – if it is your manager then speak to a trusted colleague and go higher, remember to use other healthcare professionals for support if need be.

- *Document what you have witnessed* – to whom you have reported it and ask to be informed of the response.
- *No response?* Then think of who else you can speak to and pursue the matter.

Remember, taking action is an act of bravery, by witnessing bad practice and not reporting it you are accepting this practice.

The 1988 Whistleblowing Act also protects employees who disclose that a member of staff is being bullied, harassed or discriminated against. As employees we have the right to be free of harassment, to be treated equally and not to be bullied. Equally, the organisation has a responsibility to be open, accountable and committed to treat concerns confidentially and without reprisals or victimisation.

FINAL THOUGHTS

This chapter has explored what our human rights are and how we may expect to be treated when entering a healthcare environment. It has also looked at consent, confidentiality and witnessing poor practice. As healthcare workers we all have a responsibility to ensure that people are treated equally and that we see them as partners in their care.

FURTHER READING

There are many books, articles and websites that offer more information, scenarios and answers in terms of equality, diversity and rights in healthcare. Here are some suggestions.

BOOKS

- Dimond B (2002) *Legal Aspects of Nursing* (3e). Longman, London. A book that covers a breadth of legal issues. Dimond also makes the law seem understandable by linking it into clinical scenarios.

WEBSITES

- www.doh.gov.uk/consent A good source, as it will also link you to other healthcare sites. The consent section is excellent with downloadable guides for you to use.
- www.eoc.org.uk This is the Equal Opportunities Commission website and is a good source for European and government directives, to which our organisations are accountable.

Chapter 5

CHALLENGING BEHAVIOUR

Mary Moriarty

INTRODUCTION

This chapter explores challenging behaviour and what this means in practice. Having to deal with aggressive and abusive behaviour can be extremely difficult, especially when you have a duty of care to the person who is behaving badly towards you. It can be easy to just accept a person's behaviour because *'They're always like that'*. Labelling someone as 'difficult' or 'awkward', without trying to gain an insight into why they are behaving in this way, does not help to improve their care. Ironically it may hide a real need, which they are unable to express in a way we can easily understand. Not all challenging behaviour should be viewed as negative; sometimes it can stretch us to think of different and more creative ways of approaching the way we deliver care.

'Challenging behaviour' is a term commonly used and it can mean different things to different people. It is most often identified as verbal and physical abuse. So, what does challenging behaviour mean? A simple definition for challenging behaviour could be 'any behaviour which challenges you to be calm and effective in what you do'.

BEHAVIOURS THAT ARE CHALLENGING

The following situations may also be considered challenging:

- being ignored
- demanding attention
- belittling
- invasion of space
- sarcasm
- criticism
- confusion
- constant noise.

 Challenging behaviours

List some of the behaviours that you have to deal with that you consider to be challenging.

It is important to recognise that we do not just experience challenging behaviour with patients, it can also come from relatives, carers, other staff, in fact anyone with whom we come into contact. We also have to deal with it outside work, whether it is road rage, people 'pushing in' at supermarket queues or children screaming.

It is not necessarily angry or threatening behaviour that is the most difficult to manage. If you are looking after someone who has dementia and is confused they may constantly be trying to leave the ward and it can be very difficult to relieve their distress and keep them safe.

Different people will find some behaviour more difficult or challenging than others; for example, some people find swearing very offensive while others are not bothered by it. It can be helpful to recognise the behaviours that you find the most difficult to deal with.

Consider 'what pushes your buttons'; knowing this may help you to alter your response to an incident when it occurs.

 A challenging situation

Think about a situation that you found particularly challenging. Describe the behaviour.

TRIGGERS OF CHALLENGING BEHAVIOUR

The causes of challenging behaviour will vary, but there is always a *trigger* for it. Sometimes if you know what the triggers are, challenging behaviour can be prevented. You can alter your response or perhaps you can intervene earlier to prevent a situation from escalating. Figure 5.1 illustrates a number of potential triggers.

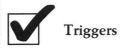 **Triggers**

Think about your challenging situation – what could have been the trigger for the person's behaviour?

YOUR REACTIONS

As situations escalate you may feel like running away or perhaps you may feel that you must stay and sort it out. This is often referred to as the 'flight or fight' experience. This is normal and happens as a result of adrenaline being produced in the body. Adrenaline has the effect of speeding up our reactions so our body prepares for physical activity. This can also reduce our capacity for rational thought and so some people have the experience of 'freezing' – not knowing what to do or say.

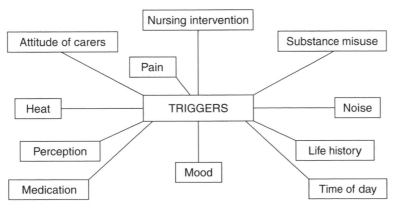

Figure 5.1   Triggers of challenging behaviour.

WHAT WAS THE CRISIS POINT?

Think what was the most difficult point in a situation you have been involved in, what was the crisis point? Again, there are thoughts and feelings that people commonly experience at this point – fear, anger, guilt, feeling unsupported and unsure of what to do. It may not have resulted in someone being physically hurt, but you may have feared that it would. Fear can be just as frightening. If you think about a horror film, it is not what you see that is always the most frightening part of the film, it is what is left to your imagination. This feeling of fear is very real and can affect you both physically and psychologically.

AFTER EXPERIENCING A CHALLENGING SITUATION

When the situation starts to calm down and recovery happens there are often some after-effects. In the short term, feelings of avoidance are normal. You may want to stay out of someone's way or in certain circumstances you may not want to go in to work. You may have intrusive thoughts, you just cannot stop thinking about it. You also are very aware of the other person and expect them to start behaving that way again. You feel 'on your guard' with them and this may make you more vigilant.

It is important to note that it can take up to 90 minutes for the adrenaline within your body to return to normal levels. During this time a person can be more easily restimulated into another crisis. As adrenaline breaks down it can have a depressing effect, so feeling low is also common. It is not just the person exhibiting the challenging behaviour who goes through these stages but also the person dealing with it and possibly other people who observe what happens.

 Managing challenging sitautions

Now think back to your situation you described earlier, how did you manage it?

SUPPORT MECHANISMS

Support is vital but it may mean different things to different people. After an incident has occurred some people will want to discuss it straight afterwards, whereas others may want to go away and calm down before they talk about it.

The important thing is that individuals are allowed to choose the support they find the most helpful.

Support does not just mean having an opportunity to talk to someone. It is also about having clear policies and procedures in place so that individuals are aware of their responsibilities when a difficulty arises. If a patient on a medical ward has a cardiac arrest the procedure is very clear, the cardiac arrest team are all aware of their own and each other's role. So the more prepared people are, the more supportive it feels. Feeling safe and knowing how to get help gives people more confidence to deal effectively with a situation.

 Support mechanisms

What policies and procedures in relation to challenging behaviour are available in your workplace?

IDENTIFYING KEY ISSUES

The key to most instances of challenging behaviour is communication. The difficulties we often encounter occur because we have not always understood someone before we have tried to get them to understand us. It is vital that the person we are dealing with knows that we have understood them correctly, so we need to communicate that to them clearly. The following points are key to effective communication:

- listen actively
- check that you have understood someone correctly – ask for more information if necessary
- resist arguing
- agree where criticism is truthful – admit failings
- be clear and honest about what you can and cannot do
- refer to others who may be able to help
- explore positive action plans.

 Key issues

What were the key issues for you regarding the incident you described?

There is no magic solution to dealing with challenging, abusive or aggressive behaviour. Your safety and the safety of others is very important.

- Request the behaviour to stop, for example '*I would like to help but I need you to stop shouting ...*'
- Keep yourself calm – be aware of voice, facial expression, eye contact, etc. – yours and the individual's.
- Be aware of exits.
- Maintain distance between you and the individual.
- Watch for changes in behaviour.
- Divert and/or distract their attention to something else.
- Take the initiative by telling the person what you want them to do – do not approach an armed assailant.
- Consider leaving the situation – the 'First Aid principle' – keep yourself safe first.

Every situation is different but the more information you have regarding individuals and their situations the more likely you will be able to respond effectively. Knowing how and when to get help will also increase your safety and your confidence.

REPORTING INCIDENTS

Incidents should be recorded and reported accurately. Make sure you know how you should report these incidents in your workplace.

 Reporting incidents

What is the procedure for recording and/or reporting incidents in your organisation?

Whatever approach you take, think about what might happen afterwards. Whether the behaviour involves a patient, relative or staff member you may have to continue working with them. Establishing and maintaining a positive relationship is something to consider when deciding on how to deal with a difficult situation.

 Planning for the future

On reflection, what could you or others have done differently to bring the situation you described earlier to a more satisfactory conclusion?

FINAL THOUGHTS

We all encounter difficulties at times, and you will continue to find that there are situations that arise that cause you to feel uncomfortable. The important thing is to realise that everyone goes through this. It can be useful to think about how you would like to be treated if you were in a similar situation, keeping in mind at the same time that we are all different. We can all be wise with hindsight and think of ways in which we could have managed things differently. It is how we can learn from these situations that helps us to be better prepared in the future.

FURTHER READING

- Stokes G and Allan B (1990) Seeking an explanation. In: G Stokes and F Goudie (eds) *Working with Dementia*. Winslow Press, Bicester.
- Smith P (1983) The assault cycle. Cited in: SG Kaplan and EG Wheeler. Survival skills for working with potentially violent clients. *Social Casework*. **64**(6): 339–46.
- Breakwell GM (1989) *Facing Physical Violence*. Routledge, London.

Chapter 6

HEALTH AND SAFETY: TIPS FOR THE WORKPLACE

Virginia Playford

INTRODUCTION

In our everyday life the ability to see, hear, smell, taste and touch alerts us to dangers and helps us to avoid them. Our memory and perceptual ability helps us to ensure our safety and to avoid harm as far as possible. If we are ill or in need of care and are admitted into a healthcare environment, we become dependent on others for our health and safety.

As individuals, we all have a part to play in ensuring that we safeguard the welfare of others and ourselves throughout our lives, both at home and at work. This chapter aims to raise awareness and develop understanding of health and safety within the workplace. It looks at the knowledge and skills needed to recognise when things are unsafe or could go wrong, how risk management is essential for a safe environment and employers' responsibilities to employees, patients, visitors and members of the public and others within the workplace.

The chapter contains eight activities, their aim is to help you focus on your practice and to raise your awareness and understanding of health and safety within your workplace.

HISTORY

For a healthy and secure workplace a number of measures have been designed to protect individuals at work. These measures are also designed to protect others, such as patients, visitors and members of the public who may be affected by work activities within the environment.

The UK was the first country in the world to pass legislation to protect the health and well-being of people at work, in the form of The Health and Morals of Apprentices Act of 1802. However, it was not until the Factory Act of 1833, when inspectors were appointed to enforce health and safety at work, that the law really became effective.

In 1970, the government appointed a commission of inquiry to conduct a review of health and safety legislation. The 1972 report of that inquiry became the basis of the Health and Safety at Work Act 1974. This Act placed broad general duties on employers, employees and others, although much of the detailed requirements are stated in additional regulations enabled by this original Act.

Most people spend a significant part of their lives at work and do not expect their health to be affected by work-related incidents. It has been estimated that in the UK alone approximately 300 people die each year as a result of work-related accidents and up to a further 2.5 million people suffer work-related ill health.

Accidents and illness cause a great deal of personal pain and suffering for individuals as well as worry and financial difficulties for their families.

Injuries and ill health at work are most commonly caused by:

- lifting, moving, carrying and other manual handling activities
- slipping, tripping and falling
- cross-infection
- being exposed to harmful substances, such as chemicals
- making contact with electricity
- various effects of fire, such as heat and smoke.

All employers, employees and the self-employed have specific legal responsibilities for health and safety at work. The Health and Safety at Work Act 1974 covers these responsibilities.

Employers must ensure that the health, safety and welfare of employees are protected so far as reasonably practicable by providing a safe system of work, competent staff and safe premises, plant and equipment. In particular, employers must:

- provide and maintain workplace systems that are safe
- deal with substances such as chemicals in a safe manner
- provide information, instruction, training and supervision
- appoint a competent person or persons to assist with health and safety
- maintain a safe and healthy workplace with the necessary welfare facilities
- provide personnel with protective equipment or clothing where necessary
- provide health and safety policies and procedures as guidance for employees
- carry out risk assessments.

Employers must also ensure that the workplace and work activities do not put employees, patients, visitors and members of the public at unnecessary risk.

 Health and safety

Using the Buzan diagram shown in Figure 6.1 complete a list of people you come into contact with during a typical working day.

All these people could be at risk of injury if the working environment is not safe.

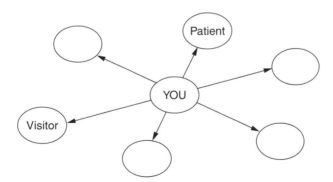

Figure 6.1 A Buzan diagram (after Buzan, 1998).

EMPLOYER DUTIES

It shall be the duty of every employer to ensure, so far as it is reasonably practicable, the health and welfare at work of all his employees.

Health and Safety at Work Act 1974 (section 2)

This means that employers must take reasonable care to protect their employees from the risk of foreseeable injury, disease or death while at work. To ensure that this is undertaken employers must be able to demonstrate that the following have been provided and are suitably maintained.

- A safe place of work, including safe entrances and exits.
- A safe system of work.
- Safe plant and equipment.
- Safe and competent fellow employees.

EMPLOYEE DUTIES

> It shall be the duty of every employee while at work to take reasonable care of health and safety of himself and other persons who may be affected by his acts and omissions while at work.
>
> Health and Safety at Work Act 1974 (section 7)

Employees have a duty to obey the reasonable instructions of their employers and to take all reasonable care in carrying out their duties. Employees also have a legal responsibility to:

- take care of their own personal health and safety at work
- take care of the health and safety of others
- co-operate with their employer in matters of health and safety
- not misuse or interfere with anything provided for health and safety purposes.

 Responsibilities

Make a list of your personal responsibilities for health and safety during one shift.

Write down how the safety of a colleague might be compromised by a work activity.

FACTORS THAT AFFECT HEALTH, SAFETY AND SECURITY AT WORK

- *Occupational* – individuals may be at risk from certain illnesses or injury because of the type of work they are doing. In the healthcare environment such risks may be caused by working with dangerous substances, needlestick injuries or suffering back problems, falls, sprains and strains.
- *Environmental* – the conditions in which people have to work may cause problems, for example inadequate space, unsuitable lighting or trailing wires and cables.
- *Human* – individuals' poor behaviour or attitude may contribute to accidents. This may include errors such as carelessness, ignorance of or not following correct policies and procedures.

 Factors affecting health and safety at work

Give one example for each of the above factors (occupational, environmental and human).

It is also worth remembering many accidents often result from a combination of human factors with faults with equipment or the workplace.

It is essential that the National Health Service, as an employer, demonstrates its commitment to the Health and Safety at Work Act 1974 by having clearly defined, up-to-date policies and procedures in order to maintain a safe and secure working environment for all.

 Who is responsible?

Find out whom has the ultimate responsibility for ensuring these policies are effective and up-to-date in your work area.

Name of individual(s):

Most countries have developed legislation to protect the health and safety of individuals at work. In the UK, employers must take the responsibility to care for and protect employees and others from the risk of injury, disease or death. A degree of responsibility is also placed on employees to take care to protect themselves and others. Employees are also responsible for ensuring their own health and safety within their workplace. It is also the duty of employees to report any problems or issues about health and safety to managers or to the named health and safety representative. The health and safety representative will be a member of the workforce who has been appointed to ensure a safe environment. They often have an interest in health and safety and should receive regular training to take responsibility for ensuring that health and safety standards are met. It is also common within healthcare that there are representatives for moving and handling, first aid and fire marshalling. These individuals are there to advise and train employees within their specific work areas. These roles are in addition to their daily work.

 Your health and safety

Write down the name of the health and safety representative for your area.

Name of health and safety representative:

RISK MANAGEMENT

An effective health and safety policy will depend upon both employers and employees successfully weighing up risk. This approach focuses on social responsibility and the need to comply with legislation.

Risk may be classified as:

- those we must take (such as walking to work, crossing the road)
- those we cannot afford to take (such as exposure to health-threatening practices)
- those we cannot afford *not* to take (such as helping someone else in an accident, breakthrough technology).

Risk management, therefore, is an essential part of our everyday activities and may be seen from different perspectives. In healthcare risk management often takes the form of 'risk assessment'. Risk assessment results from reporting incidents or near-misses, the aim of the approach being to encourage individuals to think about what could go wrong and of ways to prevent accidents occurring.

Employee expectations are far greater than in the past. If a healthcare organisation is to succeed it must consider the quality of working life. Health and safety is therefore a central part of any quality assurance process and will ultimately affect the delivery of patient care.

RISK ASSESSMENT

Risk assessment and incident reporting in the work environment is a legal requirement. It demonstrates good practice and aids in highlighting areas where training is required, as well as assisting towards quality assurance programmes. It often enables organisations to reduce the costs associated with accidents and ill health of employees. It acts as a technique for preventing accidents and ill health, by encouraging individuals to report incidents and near-misses, and encourages them to think about what could go wrong.

Risk assessments must be carried out in every workplace on activities that could cause harm. These assessments are usually completed by the named representatives for health and safety, who, understanding the task or issue being assessed, are aware of suitable safety controls and of legal requirements. The guidance of these assessments will conform to hospital policies.

The assessment process involves analysing tasks carefully to estimate the nature and level of hazard and potential risks. It is common practice for all staff to become involved with this process as the workplace and daily activities must be examined carefully. Some hazards will be obvious, others may be more difficult to identify. When carrying out a risk assessment it is necessary to identify hazards, decide who might be harmed, evaluate risks and record findings.

Risk assessment need not be overly complicated. Individuals carry out risk assessments during almost all their waking lives. When we cross the road we are able to quickly assess the risks from moving vehicles. However, in the workplace, where significant hazards and risks are present, these must be recorded and records kept. A review should always take place when changes are made and all individuals concerned informed. If new equipment is introduced it should be risk-assessed, and all staff should receive training with it before it is used. The representative who has been appointed for health and safety should keep a record of staff who attended training sessions. All staff should know where the risk assessment documentation is kept and be able to access it at any time.

Risk assessment

Locate the risk assessment policies or folder in your area for moving and handling. Look at the assessment on transferring a patient from a chair onto a bed.

Does the policy reflect practice?

WHAT ARE HAZARDS AND RISKS?

Hazards within the workplace should be removed as far as possible. Unfortunately, this is not always achievable and there is no alternative but to keep them and reduce the risk of an accident or harm being caused to individuals.

- A *hazard* is anything that has the potential to cause harm within the workplace (for example, chemicals, electricity, or falls on a wet floor).
- A *risk* is the chance, big or small, of harm actually being caused.

If we consider a simple task such as crossing the road, the *hazard* is actually the vehicles coming towards us, whereas the *risk* is the chance that we will be hit by a vehicle.

 Hazards and risks

Think of a work activity that could be classed as hazardous, which also has an element of risk for harm or illness to individuals.

Jot down your ideas here.

INCIDENT REPORTING

Reporting incidents and near-misses is the responsibility of all employees. Incident reporting should cover all areas, including assault, fire and theft. All staff should be committed to identifying and minimising risk. This may only be achieved by educating them to ensure that hazards are identified quickly and dealt with in a proactive, positive and responsive way. Reporting adverse incidents is also essential to the success of risk management. Staff should be encouraged to report and complete incident forms in order to reduce the risk of harm to employees, patients, visitors, members of the public and others.

 Incident reporting

Write down, in your own words, how you would explain to a new colleague why incidents and near-misses should be reported.

FINAL THOUGHTS

Patients and colleagues depend on us to provide a healthy, safe and secure environment. Government legislation requires that employers have guidelines and regulations, in the form of policies and procedures, in place. For these to be effective all employees need education and training. All staff should work together to raise awareness of hazards and the reporting of incidents or near-misses.

Both employers and employees are obliged to comply with government legislation by undertaking suitable risk assessments. The findings of these risk assessments should be used to ensure a positive proactive approach to safeguarding all individuals, including patients, visitors and members of the public, who may be affected by workplace activities.

FURTHER READING

- Buzan T and Buzan B (1998) *The Mindmap Book*. BBC Books, London.
- Clarke P and Jones J (1998) *Brigden's Operation Department Practice*. Churchill Livingstone, London.
- Health and Safety Executive (1988) *Essentials of Health & Safety at Work*. Health & Safety Executive, London.

- Chartered Institute of Environmental Health (1998) *Health & Safety First Principles.* Chadwick House Group Ltd, London. This is a very good book. It has all the basic principles of health and safety, and is easy to read. Available from the Chartered Institute of Environmental Health, www.cieh.org
- Health and Safety Executive (2000) *Management of Health & Safety at Work Regulations 1999.* www.hsebooks.co.uk
- NHS Executive (1996) *Risk Management in the NHS.* Department of Health, London.

Chapter 7

MATHEMATICAL SKILLS FOR HEALTHCARE

Sally Ballard

INTRODUCTION

This chapter looks at a range of mathematical skills and how they apply to healthcare. The word *mathematical* rather than *numerical* is used deliberately as it is often numbers that scare people. As soon as some people see a formula they think 'maths' and start to worry. Numbers are shorthand for mathematical ideas, such as volume, speed and dimension, and it is these ideas that this chapter focuses on. If you have a solid understanding of the underpinning ideas, this will give you the confidence to develop your skills further.

This chapter covers:

- the mathematical ideas that underpin the human body
- the metric system
- recording measurements in practice, and understanding the significance of such recordings
- visual and graphical representation of the human condition.

You will see that this chapter deliberately avoids the use of formulae and numbers much of the time. There are existing texts that cover these areas (*see* Further Reading at the end of the chapter). This chapter has been written as a forerunner to such texts. The aim is to build your confidence. Unfortunately, too many people have a poor opinion of their mathematical ability and this need not be the case.

MATHEMATICAL IDEAS THAT UNDERPIN THE HUMAN BODY

How does 'maths' apply in healthcare? Very simply, because the human body may be described as a system of weights and measures, you can describe a person as a series of volumes, lengths, weights, pressures, temperatures and so on. Similarly, what you observe happening to someone over the course of time may be described in mathematical terms. There are criticisms to this approach to healthcare (some describe it as a *reductionist* view, which reduces the person to a series of numbers) but a certain amount of mathematical observation is essential in monitoring the well-being of a person.

 An example of a mathematical idea underpinning the human body

What did you drink for breakfast this morning?

Put your answer here.

If you have written 'a cup of tea' or 'a glass of orange juice' this is a perfectly good answer. However, an alternative answer would be this:

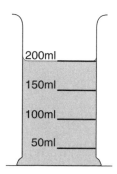

You may not readily think of this reply to the above question, but it is a correct answer. Representing your cup of tea as a volume of liquid is a *mathematical* way of describing your drink this morning, whereas the phrase 'a cup of tea' or 'a glass of orange' is a *literal* description. You will find in healthcare that you have to be able to describe a person's well-being and behaviour in both mathematical and literal ways.

As previously stated, the human body may be thought of as a series of volumes and measures. These are mathematical ways of describing a person. Look at the following description.

What am I?

This object weighs about 90 kilograms (kg) and, when laid out on the ground, measures 180 centimetres (cm) in length and 50 cm in width. It contains roughly 50 litres (L) of fluid. Two litres of fluid enter it and leave it on a regular basis. One end is spherical in shape with a circumference of 60 cm. The other end is split into two sections. The surface area of each of these sections is 300 cm².

Answer – an adult male!

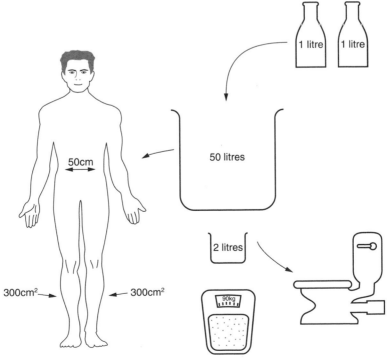

Many measurements may be used when describing a person's well-being. For example, a person's weight is a quick way of describing how well a person appears to be eating (and their health generally). Someone who has gained or lost weight may have a health condition that needs investigating. Perhaps the best known example of this is with newborn babies. Throughout their first year of life babies are weighed regularly to check that they are growing at an acceptable rate.

The main point to take in is that the numbers that you see recorded in patients' notes, and that you too will record, are simply a shorthand description of the human body.

THE METRIC SYSTEM

All measurements need to be taken by use of an agreed scale. Weight (or more accurately *mass*), volume and length now need to be measured using the metric system. Those of you born after 1980 may wonder what else there is, but those of us born before 1980 may still be wrestling with the metric system because we were brought up with a different system (that consisted of measures such as *pints*, *miles* and *stones!*).

To sense how hard it can be to think in a different system, just imagine that the UK has decided to switch to the euro as its currency. You now have to think of all prices and values using euros instead of pounds and pence. How much will a house cost? What is the price of petrol? What will you expect to earn per hour?

It is possible to use conversion tables between the imperial system and the metric system, but we have chosen not to include these here. The bottom line is that all measurements now need to use the metric system. So you need to be confident with it. Equipment you use will be calibrated in metric units. The harder part is learning to think, and therefore estimating, in metric.

The remainder of this section will recall the metric system. Just before you skip this because you are already confident, have a go at the following questions. If you are uncertain of some of the answers, you may need to read it!

Question	Answer
How many millilitres (mL) are in a litre (L)?	There are 1000 mL in a L.
Which is heavier – a milligram (mg) or a microgram (mcg or μg)?	A milligram is heavier.
What is the relationship between metres (m) and kilometres (km)?	1000 metres = 1 km

Table 7.1 Metric units in common use

	Unit (abbreviation)	Other units (abbreviation)
Weight or mass	gram (gm)	kilogram (kg); milligram (mg); microgram (mcg or μg)
Volume	litre (L)	kilolitre (kL); millilitre (ml); microlitre (mcL)
Length	metre (m)	kilometre (km); centimetre (cm); millimetre (mm)

The metric units you are most likely to use or come across are shown in Table 7.1.

Some of these units should be familiar to you, for example in a shop produce is labelled in grams (g), kilograms (kg) and litres (L). You may already see a pattern emerging in Table 7.1 above, the same prefixes are used each time. This was deliberate when the metric system was designed. What you need to understand is the relationship between each unit, for example between a gram and a kilogram, fortunately they follow patterns, which again was deliberate in the metric design.

WEIGHT

Let us look at the relationship between grams and kilograms. Say a baby elephant weighs 1 kg and a mouse weighs 1 g. You need to pile up 1000 mice to weigh the same as one baby elephant.

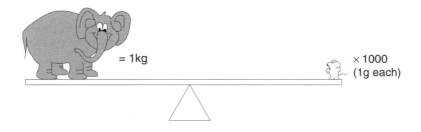

Introducing numbers, here you can say that 1 kg = 1000 g. This is a numerical way of describing the relationship.

A point to take from the previous illustration is that 1000 g and 1 kg are identical in weight. By being the same you can use either unit to describe the weight of something. For example, a 1 kg bag of sugar may be described as weighing 1000 g. These two expressions are an identical weight, and in this case they describe the same object (the bag of sugar). However, objects with identical weights may not be the same in other ways. You can appreciate how much more space the mice would take up and how many more of them there would be compared to the elephant. Remember to keep in mind what we are actually describing – not the animals shown but an object or substance that feels 1 kg (or 1000 g) 'heavy'. Ultimately, the numbers on this page relate to a physical property or dimension that you can sense. People lose their way with maths because numbers on a page become divorced from the real world.

Now let us look at the relationship between grams and milligrams. Using a similar idea let us say that our mouse still weighs 1 g and an ant weighs 1 milligram (mg). You need to pile up 1000 ants to weigh the same as the mouse.

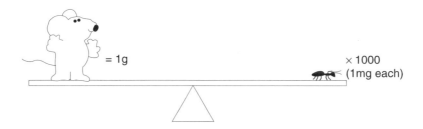

Therefore 1 g = 1000 mg.

You might see a pattern emerging. If a microgram (mcg or μg) is lighter than a milligram (mg), can you guess what the relationship between the two would be? The answer is that there are 1000 mcg (μg) in a milligram (or 1 mg = 1000 mcg or μg). Part of the difficulty at this point is trying to comprehend something that weighs as little as a microgram. Again let us say a bacterium weighs 1 mcg (μg). You need to pile up 1000 bacteria to equal the weight of one ant.

In healthcare which units of weight are you most likely to use?

The answer is kilograms (weights of people) and grams (weights of objects such as swabs used in the operating theatre). You are unlikely to have to measure in milligrams and micrograms. You would need scientific scales to get this level of accuracy. One area where you would be likely to encounter such small weights would be drug administration. Drugs are usually measured in mg or mcg (μg). If you think how light these units are (particularly in relation to how heavy you are) you get a sense of how powerful drugs are to the human body.

Using the metric system

- Familiarise yourself with the metric units of weight (or more accurately *mass*) and their abbreviations. The largest one presented here is a kilogram (kg), the smallest a microgram (mcg or μg). There are heavier and even lighter units, but in healthcare you are unlikely to encounter them.

- Think about the relationship between the units of weight – kilograms, grams, milligrams and micrograms. Each time 1000 of the smaller units equals the larger unit. Mathematical knowledge includes ideas about relationships. It is the relationship between the units that you need to grasp at this stage.

- The units of weight we have looked at relate to a physical property in the real world. In this case they relate to the heaviness you experience when asked to handle an object or substance. Try holding certain objects at home (such as a 1 kg bag of sugar) to get a sense of their weight.

VOLUME

Now you have the units for measuring weight, let us move on to volume. We will start with a base unit for volume of a litre (L). The units for measuring volume were given earlier in Table 7.1. Can you suggest what the relationship between the units of volume might be? (Clue – look at the prefixes kilo-, milli- and micro-.) (*See* Table 7.2.)

Table 7.2 Relationship between units of volume

Unit of volume	*Relationship*
Kilolitre (kL)	1 kL = 1000 litres (L)
Litre (L)	1 L = 1000 millilitres (mL)
Millilitre (mL)	1 mL = 1000 microlitres (μL)*
Microlitre (μL)	1 μL = 1000 nanolitres (nL)*

* You are unlikely to come across either unit in practice.

It is essential to ground your understanding of volume to some real examples. Volume describes the space that a fluid occupies. What does one litre of fluid look like? Typically, supermarkets sell juice or milk in 1 L cartons. A car petrol tank may hold 40 L of petrol. Does this conjure up any sense of space for you? (Often it does not as you cannot see the petrol tank that you are filling.) It is worth having some sense of what 1 L versus 1 mL of fluid looks like. In healthcare you may be asked to estimate how much urine a patient has passed, or how much blood they have lost in a nosebleed.

LENGTH

We will use a base unit for length measurement of one metre (m).

 Units of length

Construct your own table showing the units of length measurement and examples of when you might encounter them – both at work and in everyday life. What is the relationship between the units?

You may have some trouble with the centimetre. It has a different prefix from the examples we have looked at so far. It is a common unit of length so you need to know its relationship to a metre. Appendix I contains a table for you to compare your answer.

You may also hear metric units described as 'SI units'. 'SI' stands for 'Système International d'Unités'. The metric system originates from 1790 and the French Academy of Science. It was designed as a completely new system of units to be used throughout the world. If you are interested in a brief overview of the metric system, try the following website: www.hlalapansi.demon.co.uk/Metric/. It is technical, but gives you a brief history of the metric system and a table of all the prefixes.

Metric dimensions

How well do you know your vital statistics in the metric system? Record the following about yourself:

Weight _____

Height _____

Head circumference _____

Calf circumference _____

Your fluid intake _____ (on an average day)

RECORDING MEASUREMENTS IN PRACTICE

In practice you will use some of the SI units given in this section, though probably not all of them. Litres, millilitres, grams, kilograms, metres and millimetres are common units that you will encounter as you care for patients.

 Measurement in practice

Can you think of examples in healthcare where you will use the above metric units?

(*For example*, weekly weighing of babies at the health clinic.)

RECORDING MEASUREMENTS IN PATIENT RECORDS

So far we have considered the types of mathematical ideas you will encounter in healthcare. By far the most common are ones concerning dimensions, such as volumes, weights and lengths. We have also revised metric dimensions because you will be expected to work with these units (even if you do not readily think in metric). You will then be expected to record measurements in patient notes.

To look at this area it is easiest to follow an example. A very common chart you will encounter is the fluid balance chart. This is a record of fluids taken into the body (typically through drinking) and the fluids excreted (typically through passing urine). Under normal circumstances the body is able to keep itself in balance. It does not get too diluted (too much fluid) or too concentrated (not enough fluid). This process of keeping the body in balance is called 'homeostasis'. The body is able to tell when it is getting too diluted. A dilute state prompts the kidneys to produce more urine to get rid of the excess fluid. You will have noticed how, on a night out to the pub, you visit the toilet more frequently as the evening wears on. Hence the well-known phrase 'you rent beer rather than buy it'! Homeostasis can be upset if you drink too little or too much or if you expel too much or too little fluid.

A fluid balance chart is used to record, and therefore monitor, the amount of fluid a person is taking in and passing out. Each recording on the chart represents a volume of fluid the person has consumed or expelled. We do not necessarily drink from fixed-volume containers. You can probably state that you drank a cup of tea for breakfast but you would not necessarily know the volume you consumed. So to be able to complete the fluid balance chart you need to know typical volumes of the fluids we drink.

Take a look at various cups, mugs and bottles that people drink from. Do you know how much fluid they hold? Commercial containers of water are labelled. Typically, a can contains 330 mL and a small bottle 500 mL.

In everyday life we do not have to be too exact about these measurements, but when a person is unwell the precise volumes become important.

What about the volumes that people expel? The biggest volume of fluid you expel is in the form of urine. Do people urinate into measured canisters? Not usually, but in a healthcare setting patients may be asked to do just this – to urinate into a pot or bottle so that you can measure their output. Alternatively, patients may have a catheter device, which means their urine is collected into a bag. Such urine bags are usually calibrated, making measurement much easier.

The next section explains how to record volumes on a fluid chart, and how to make sense of the completed chart.

 Use the following description to complete the fluid balance chart.

Chris Robinson (Hospital number 9876) is a frail 85-year-old gentleman. He lives alone. He has been neglecting himself since his wife died last year. He was admitted to hospital on 5 June 2003. In hospital you have been asked to monitor his fluid balance for 48 hours to see whether he is drinking enough. Throughout the day you keep an eye on Chris. He drinks one cup of tea at breakfast, declines a morning drink, and then has one after his lunch. He is asleep during the afternoon. He drinks another cup after supper, and accepts a cup of hot milk just before bed.

FLUID BALANCE CHART

Patient hospital no. 9876
Patient surname Robinson
Patient first name Chris

Date	Intake (in millilitres)			Output (in millilitres)	
5,6,03	Description	Intravenous	By mouth	Urine	Other
		Volume	Volume		
Time		Record at time completed			
Midnight					
1					
2					
3					
4					
5					
6					
7					
8	Cup of tea		150		
9					
10					
11					
12					
13					
14					
15					
16					
17					
18					
19					
20					
21					
22					
23					
	TOTALS				
	24 hr. Intake			24 hr. Output	

24 hour Balance

The previous description tells you Chris's fluid intake. An example of a fluid balance chart is also given. Before completing this, however, we will have to make an assumption about the volume of fluid held by an average teacup. Let us say it is 150 mL.

We now total the intake column. We have calculated that Chris has drunk a total of 600 mL today. To have some sense of how good or bad this quantity is, we need to know how much a person typically drinks in a day. Textbooks quote 2 L as a recommended fluid intake for an average adult. However, older people tend to drink less than this. It would be reasonable to expect Chris to drink something like 1200 mL per day given his age. Compare this to Chris's fluid balance chart and you can see he is not drinking enough.

Chris allows you to monitor his fluid output during the day (although he does not like you accompanying him to the toilet much). He uses a urine bottle on each visit, which he lets you measure. The urine outputs are as follows:

- Before breakfast 300 mL
- After lunch 250 mL
- Early evening 300 mL

(We will assume that he does not need to urinate overnight.)

Return to the fluid balance chart and complete the output column, including a total output for the day.

You should have a total fluid output of 850 mL. Chris's intake was 600 mL. What sense do you make of this?

Overall Chris has expelled more fluid than he has taken in. This may be described as having a *negative* fluid balance. The fluid balance is calculated by subtracting the output from the input.

As the output is the larger figure, you have a negative balance. For one day, this is not too much of a worry, but if it continues Chris will dehydrate. He will slowly reduce the amount of fluid in his body. This will lead to problems such as low blood pressure.

Appendix II contains the completed fluid balance chart for Chris. You may wish to compare it to yours.

If this was your own home and Chris was your father, you probably would not record this information. However, in your caring capacity you need to keep a written record that you are monitoring Chris's fluid balance. You need not actually record it on a chart. You could simply write down the numbers

Date	\multicolumn{3}{c}{FLUID BALANCE CHART}	Patient hospital no. ....7878.... Patient surname ....Robinson.... Patient first name ....Chris....		
Date	\multicolumn{3}{c}{Intake (in millilitres)}		\multicolumn{2}{c}{Output (in millilitres)}

Date	Description	Intravenous	By mouth	Urine	Other
5,6,03		Volume	Volume		
Time		Record at time completed			
Midnight					
1					
2					
3					
4					
5					
6					
TOTALS			600	850	
	24 hr. Intake	600		24 hr. Output 850	

24 hour Balance Intake minus Output
= −250 ml

in his notes, but the fluid balance chart provides a summary of this information. Numerical ('the numbers') representation is a very convenient shorthand at times.

If you are nervous of the numbers it is important to remember what they represent. In this case they represent the volumes of fluid that the person is taking into and expelling out from the body. This fluid is dispersed in cells, blood and linings throughout the body.

In practice you will probably perform some part of recording someone's fluid balance. You are unlikely to be present the whole 24 hours to see the totals, but you need to ensure you complete your part accurately.

This section has presented one specific example of recording measurements in patient records. You will come across many others in healthcare. A final thought before we leave this topic. We have looked at recording measurements on a fluid balance chart for Chris Robinson. We have done this for him. What if Chris kept his own fluid balance chart? This would involve him in his care and might help him to understand the importance of drinking enough fluid. You might want to consider how you would explain to Chris about filling in a fluid balance chart.

VISUAL AND GRAPHICAL PRESENTATION OF THE HUMAN CONDITION

We have just looked at recording numbers on a fluid balance chart. This involved some manipulation of numbers. Another way of representing measurements is in a visual, or graphical, form. The phrase 'a picture paints a thousand words' is apt here. You can convey information quickly by use of visual techniques. Graphs and bar charts are examples of visual presentation of information.

How could we represent the fluid balance exercise in a visual form? There are probably a number of alternatives, but one way would be to colour in two containers representing fluid intake and fluid output. For example:

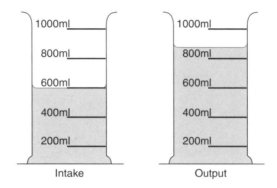

	Intake		Output

This visual chart conveys the same information as the fluid balance chart. You might like to consider whether you find this type of chart easier to understand, just as earlier we considered learning styles. Some people understand visual information more easily than numerical information.

Measurements concerning people's well-being may be recorded in a visual form. The best-known example is the observation chart, which includes temperature, pulse, respiration and blood pressure. We will look at an example, concentrating on the pulse.

 Visual presentation of information

Janet Lemcke (Hospital number 1234) is a 25-year-old lady. She is on two-hourly observations (this means you have been asked to check her pulse, blood pressure and temperature every two hours). Today is 12 December 2003. For the last 12 hours her pulse has been:

- 10 am   72 beats per minute (bpm)
- 12 noon   74 bpm
- 2 pm   70 bpm
- 4 pm   98 bpm
- 6 pm   110 bpm
- 8 pm   126 bpm

Record these pulse readings on the observation chart provided (Appendix III) Do not forget to label the chart with patient details and with the time of the recordings. What has happened to Janet's pulse over the 12 hours?

Appendix IV contains the completed observation chart for Janet. You may wish to compare it to yours.

Janet's pulse has been rising. How can you tell this from the observation chart? Because the line rises. However, it is essential to have the scales along the axes to confirm this. Essentially, this means that you must label both the vertical and horizontal lines to confirm the units you are using. Look again at the list of pulses in the original 'Activity' and compare this with the observation chart. Which do you find easier to understand? Does the rise in pulse leap out at you from both the text and the chart? The observation chart is a visual representation of Janet's condition. The beauty of visual representation is that it can be easier to identify *trends* over time.

To elicit some sense of how 'good' or 'bad' Janet's pulse is, you need to know the average pulse of an adult. An adult pulse is typically between 60 and 100 beats per minute. So, another comment you can make is that since 6 pm her pulse has been above normal.

Look at another form of visual presentation of information. This graph represents 'David West' who is 38 years old and is 170 cm tall.

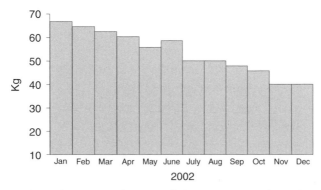

The vertical scale is labelled in kilograms, so the chart is about weight. The chart shows that David has lost weight over the past 12 months. Do you know what a person of David's height (170 cm) should weigh? About 65 kg. So, you may say that David has lost weight and is now below average weight for his height. You would need to know more about David to make any other comments. He may have been dieting for 12 months and his plan was to lose weight. Alternatively, he may have been eating normally, which may suggest a health problem that needs investigating.

Graphical or visual charts are often used in healthcare to show trends over time. You need to feel confident that you can understand such charts, and that you can complete them accurately if asked to do so.

> Always bear in mind that the information from a chart is limited in what it can tell you, it is only one piece of information. You may need to put together a number of pieces of information to gain an understanding about someone's well-being. In the example concerning Janet's pulse, you can say that her pulse has been rising and is now above a normal level. To say any more you need more information.

FINAL THOUGHTS

In this chapter we have looked at some of the mathematical ideas that will be encountered in healthcare. We have deliberately stayed away from numbers, formulae and calculations at this stage. They can be offputting, and worry people too early on. The aim has been to give you more confidence about maths. Mathematical techniques help you to describe or record events in the real world. One thought to arm yourself with through your studies is this: if colleagues blind you with numbers, ask them to draw a diagram to illustrate what they are trying to tell you. It may not be the easiest of diagrams, but there should be a way, without lots of numbers, of explaining their point.

We hope you now feel less anxious about the mathematical skills and ideas you need for healthcare practice. Below are listed some mathematical areas you might want to move on to when you are ready:

- metric conversions (for example, how to convert grams to kilograms)
- drug calculations
- fractions, decimals, percentages (how to convert a fraction to a decimal and a percentage, and understanding what these represent)
- using bar charts, pie charts and graphs to convey information
- simple statistics (for example, what the word *average* means).

FURTHER READING

- Dison N (1997) *Simplified Drugs and Solutions for Health Care Professionals* (11e). Mosby, London. A comprehensive workbook covering a range of topics (decimals and fractions through to paediatric drug calculations). It looks mathematical, but does relate calculations to practice. Be careful. As it is American it includes imperial measures and their conversion to metric.
- Eastaway R and Wyndham J (1998) *Why Do Buses Come in Threes? The Hidden Mathematics of Everyday Life.* Robson Books, London. An easy-to-read book about the maths that surrounds us. It has chapters entitled 'How do you explain a coincidence?' and 'How can I win without cheating?' This is a general interest book about mathematical ideas. It is not directly related to healthcare.
- Gatford J and Anderson R (1998) *Nursing Calculations* (5e). Churchill Livingstone, London. A very useful 'question and answer' book, which takes you through all the main drug calculations (solutions, injections) as well as revising fractions, decimals, etc. It looks mathematical, so may be a little offputting at this stage.

APPENDIX 1

METRIC UNITS OF LENGTH MEASUREMENT AND THEIR RELATIONSHIPS

Unit of length	Relationship
Kilometre (km)	1 km = 1000 metres
Metre (m)	1 m = 1000 millimetres and 1 m = 100 centimetres
Centimetre (cm)	1 cm = 10 millimetres
Millimetre (mm)	1 mm = 1000 micrometres*
Micrometre (μm)	(1 μm = 1000 nanometres)*

* You are unlikely to come across either unit in practice.

APPENDIX II

CHRIS ROBINSON'S COMPLETED FLUID BALANCE CHART

FLUID BALANCE CHART		Patient hospital no. 9876 Patient surname Robinson Patient first name Chris			
Date 5,6,03	Intake (in millilitres)			Output (in millilitres)	
	Description	Intravenous	By mouth	Urine	Other
		Volume	Volume		
Time		Record at time completed			
Midnight					
1					
2					
3					
4					
5					
6					
7					
8	Cup of tea		150	300	
9					
10					
11					
12	Cup of tea		150		
13				250	
14					
15					
16					
17	Cup of tea		150		
18				300	
19					
20					
21	Cup of milk		150		
22					
23					
	TOTALS		600	850	
	24 hr. Intake 600			24 hr. Output 850	

24 hour Balance Intake minus Output
= −250 ml

APPENDIX III

OBSERVATION CHART

OBSERVATION CHART		Patient hospital no. . . . . Patient surname . . . . Patient first name . . . .

Year . . . .

Date											
Time											

Pulse	150										
	140										
	130										
	120										
	110										
	100										
	90										
	80										
	70										
	60										
	50										
	45										
	40										
	35										
	30										
	25										
	20										
	15										
	10										
	5										

Appendix iv

Janet lemcke's completed observation chart

	OBSERVATION CHART			Patient hospital no.	1234				
				Patient surname	Lemcke				
				Patient first name	Janet				

Year 2003

Date		12/12	12/12	12/12	12/12	12/12	12/12				
Time		10⁰⁰	12⁰⁰	14⁰⁰	16⁰⁰	18⁰⁰	20⁰⁰				

Pulse

150
140
130
120
110
100
90
80
70
60
50
45
40
35
30
25
20
15
10
5

Chapter 8

APPLICATION OF SCIENCE TO HEALTHCARE

Nigel Conway and Paul Ong

INTRODUCTION

This chapter aims to help you to gain an understanding of the importance of scientific knowledge to clinical practice. It makes use of theory relating to temperature control and regulation. This will, in turn, illustrate how knowledge may be applied to your practice. A number of questions are asked and each of these is explored in more depth as you read through the text. There are several activities for you to complete. You may be able to complete some of them straightaway, whereas you may need to find information to complete others. Make use of the spaces provided for your own thoughts and notes. Table 8.1 introduces some relevant terminology for this chapter.

Think about the following question. How many times have you used a cold flannel to bring down either your own or someone else's temperature?

Many actions that we carry out as individuals, parents or carers are often referred to as being 'common sense or knowledge'. Often, this notion of 'common sense or knowledge' is taken for granted and we do not consider the theoretical principles behind it. Consequently, it is easy to take things at face value. This chapter aims to look behind this 'common sense' or 'face value'

Table 8.1   Some key words

Key words	Definition
Thermogenesis	Heat produced by a cell
Basal metabolic rate (BMR)	The energy needed by the human body to exist on a purely essential level, energy required by the vital organs.
Hypothalamus	The human body version of a thermostat, found in the centre of the brain, helps to regulate temperature
Joule	The amount of energy given off by food

approach to care and to make sense of the scientific knowledge that underpins many of our actions.

In order to be more effective carers we need clear understanding of *why* we do what we do. This must be derived from an 'evidence base', a term often used to support actions that are taken when deciding the most effective approach to care.

Evidence-based practice can be defined as 'a consensus of scientific opinion based on research'.

AN EXAMPLE

A health carer is looking after a patient, Mr Pinkerton. Mr Pinkerton has a wound infection.

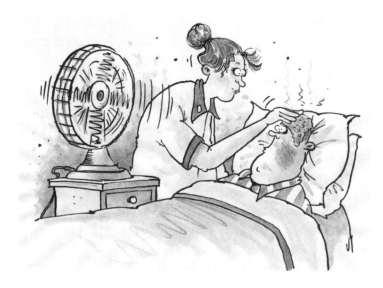

Mr Pinkerton calls the carer over and says he is feeling hot. He looks very flushed and is perspiring. He tells the carer that he feels really uncomfortable because he is so hot. The carer responds by telling Mr Pinkerton not to worry, whilst removing a blanket and asking him to take off his pyjama top. The carer also turns a fan on and applies a cold, wet flannel to Mr Pinkerton's forehead.

 Controlling temperature

Take 10 minutes to think about why these actions were carried out and jot down your ideas.

Now let us go step-by-step through the theoretical basis of why this health carer carried out these actions.

 Be cautious about taking anything at face value.

HOW DO SCIENTIFIC PRINCIPLES AFFECT PRACTICE?

A high temperature (pyrexia) is probably the symptom most commonly associated with illness. There are a number of traditional care practices adopted by health carers to manage high or low temperature.

 Temperature management

Think through the concept of temperature management.

Ask yourself the following questions and jot down some notes.

- What is heat?
- What is metabolic rate?

- What factors influence basal metabolic rate (BMR)?
- What factors influence body temperature?
- How is body temperature measured?
- Where is body temperature measured?
- What is the normal measurement for body temperature?
- How does the body regulate body temperature?
- What are the mechanisms of heat exchange?

Now that you have completed the activity let us reflect on the questions and explore some of the matters related to them.

WHAT IS HEAT?

Heat is energy and energy production in cells arises from their internal activity. This activity is referred to as 'cellular metabolism', the scientific term for this heat production is 'thermogenesis'.

WHAT IS METABOLIC RATE?

Metabolic rate is the *total* heat production of the body. This includes heat production from cells (through chemical reactions) and mechanical or physical work of the body.

WHAT FACTORS INFLUENCE BASAL METABOLIC RATE?

The energy that the body needs to exist on a purely 'essential level' is referred to as the 'basal metabolic rate' (BMR). Heat energy comes from the food we eat (carbohydrates, fats, proteins, vitamins, minerals and water) and through the processes of physical and chemical digestion.

 Heat and metabolic rate

Now that you are more aware of heat and metabolic rate can you think of five ways in which temperature can be raised within the body?

The amount of energy that is given off by different foods is measured in Joules (J). In reality this measurement is extremely small, so in healthcare we tend to measure energy values in kilo Joules (kJ). One thousand Joules (1000 J) equals one kilo Joule (1 kJ) (*see* Chapter 7).

 Heat energy

Try to find out the values of heat energy given off by the following food types. Try looking for this information in an anatomy and physiology book.

- Carbohydrates
- Fats
- Proteins
- Alcohol

WHAT FACTORS INFLUENCE BODY TEMPERATURE?

Your notes may include any of the following: time of day (lowest during sleep); exercise; exposure to variation in external temperature; disease.

 Each of these examples could be explored further in order to find out why and how they affect temperature. By asking more and more questions about such things health carers are able to build on previous knowledge and should also be able to apply this knowledge to their practice.

HOW IS BODY TEMPERATURE MEASURED?

You have probably identified a number of ways that you have either used personally or seen others use. This could include a number of different thermometers, ranging from clinical thermometers (placed onto the patient's skin, forehead), mercury thermometers (not used in hospitals now because of the danger of mercury poisoning) or electronic devices.

WHERE IS BODY TEMPERATURE MEASURED?

You may have identified that the body temperature may be taken either externally or internally, in a number of different anatomical sites. These may include orally, rectally, tympanically (ear), skin (forehead) or perhaps under the axilla (armpit).

External body temperature measurement is referred to as 'peripheral temperature' (away from the centre of the body). Effectively, this means the skin and it is greatly influenced by the external environment. Internal body temperature is referred to as 'core temperature' (central to the body). This temperature is kept constant through metabolism and the body's internal regulatory processes. Illness or a breakdown of the normal internal regulatory processes influences core temperature.

 Temperature readings

You will find that there is a variation in temperature readings between peripheral and core anatomical sites. By using books in the Further Reading list, at the end of this chapter, identify what the normal temperature readings are for the following.

- Peripheral temperature
- Core temperature

Other methods of temperature measurement include the use of wire probes. These methods tend to be used more on critically ill or unconscious patients. They are commonly placed directly onto the skin or inserted into the rectum and connected to electronic monitors (often used in intensive care units or operating theatres).

WHAT IS THE NORMAL BODY TEMPERATURE MEASUREMENT?

We must remember that body temperature varies from individual to individual for many reasons, some of which you have already identified. Other reasons could include poor health. The most important point here is that we are interested in what is the individual patient's normal temperature. This reading is often referred to as the 'baseline' temperature and all subsequent readings are compared directly to it. For most people, this temperature is approximately 37 degrees Celsius (37°C).

Armed with the results from this question we can then go on to explore the reasons for this (that is, why does the patient have a high or low temperature?) and take appropriate action to resolve the problem.

Consider the following questions.

- What is going on inside the body (chemically or metabolically)?
- Are there any external environmental issues? (Does the patient have too few or too many blankets? Is the patient breathing medical gas? Is the patient next to a draught/heater?)
- Is the body's regulatory system (hormonal or behavioural) affecting the patient's temperature?

 An example of a medical gas is oxygen. A point worth noting is that medical gases are extremely cold and dry. Medical gases may cool patients down as they breathe them.

HOW DOES THE BODY REGULATE TEMPERATURE?

You have probably come up with a list of signs or symptoms for this. This may include shivering, sweating or colour. Let us think about this a bit more. If we were to think about what regulates the central heating in a house we would eventually identify the 'thermostat'. The thermostat is usually found on a wall in the hallway and may be adjusted manually to suit your particular needs. The human body also has a 'thermostat' that enables it to adjust its temperature. This human version is known as the 'hypothalamus', which is located in the centre of the brain and makes use of other body systems, including the nervous system, circulatory system and hormonal (endocrine) system, in order to communicate with the rest of the body.

The main role of the hypothalamus is to keep the body's core temperature at the optimum level for normal cellular activity. This in turn ensures health is maintained by allowing specialist cells, tissues, organs and systems to function appropriately.

Put simply, if the body temperature is too high the hypothalamus will initiate cooling measures (sweating, vasodilation) and if the body temperature is too low it will initiate internal heat production by increasing 'thermogenesis' (cellular metabolism).

Clearly, the hypothalamus is the 'nerve centre' in terms of temperature control. However, it is only able to act in a 'supervisory way', co-ordinating and influencing other parts of the body in order to affect the body's temperature. This introduces the notion of how one part of the body has to work as part of a 'team effort' in order to maintain normal body functions or, in this case, normal temperature. This interplay of processes within the body, between anatomical sites and physiological responses, is often referred to as a 'dynamic process'.

 In teamwork any number of errors may occur, such as communication problems, poor health of one or more members of the team, power struggles, outside influences, etc. The same analogy may be applied to body functions, which is why we must always be cautious of taking things at face value.

As another analogy, think of the hypothalamus as the conductor of a small orchestra.

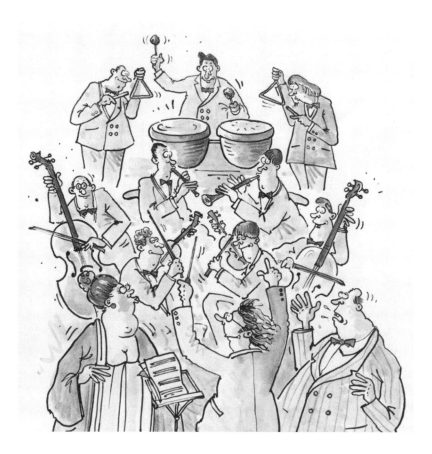

As the conductor, the hypothalamus has a 'baton' that it wields feverishly in order to maintain the flow. It is therefore able to select specific instruments or actions to co-ordinate and influence other parts of the body.

For example, the violins (peripheral veins) are situated close to the front (or surface) and will decrease or increase pitch (diameter) in order to preserve or encourage emotional feelings (heat retention or loss from the circulating blood). The *fat* opera singers represent another layer situated between them and the front (or surface), helping to reduce the pitch and outpouring of emotion (prevent heat loss, insulation).

The percussionist, right at the back (autonomic nervous system) bangs away, his beats building up (increasing the release of hormones, noradrenaline) and the pace of the music (heat production).

The wind instruments, located behind the violins, create a chill (shivering, rapid contraction of skeletal muscle, hairs stand on end trapping a layer of air on the skin surface for further insulation).

The cellos (thyroid gland) reverberate rhythmically, arms moving passionately creating a depth to the music (releasing thyroxin and increasing cellular metabolism).

A triangle chimes at the back, slowing the other instruments (sweating, cooling effect of evaporation).

WHAT ARE THE MECHANISMS OF HEAT EXCHANGE?

You may have come up with the following:

- conduction
- convection
- radiation
- evaporation.

 Heat exchange

For each of the following list three points specific to each of the mechanisms of heat exchange.

- Conduction

- Convection

- Radiation

- Evaporation

Let us now put some of this knowledge into a more practical example that you are likely to encounter.

HOW DOES AN INFECTION INFLUENCE THE BODY'S TEMPERATURE?

An infection has the effect of changing the setting of the 'thermostat' (the hypothalamus) to a higher value. The body will respond by adjusting its 'core temperature' to this new setting. In order to meet this new demand some time may pass. This helps explain why people with high temperatures can feel cold and start shivering. Mechanisms to save and generate heat will begin (vasodilation, increased metabolism). These responses will continue until the new setting is reached.

Once the body or the treatment has dealt with the infection the set-point of the thermostat (hypothalamus) will fall back to its original setting. It is usually at this point that patients complain of fever and sweat profusely as the body initiates cooling processes to bring the temperature down.

FINAL THOUGHTS

Think back to the original scenario, Mr Pinkerton was perspiring, the carer removed the blanket and his pyjama top, turned on a fan and placed a cool, wet flannel on Mr Pinkerton's forehead.

We can see now that evaporation, convection, radiation and conduction all played a part in controlling Mr Pinkerton's temperature. We can also appreciate that a number of internal responses are taking place within Mr Pinkerton's body. In essence, what we have now is a theoretical basis that underpins the carer's actions.

By going through the process of temperature regulation it becomes apparent that carers looking after patients with a high temperature should consider a number of possible causes. By thinking through the possible causes, carers will be able to initiate an appropriate response. This may include informing others as well as taking a degree of responsibility for immediate delivery of care.

By approaching healthcare in this way, carers are making use of underpinning knowledge or, more specifically, evidence derived from a scientific background. Thus their practice is influenced by science and has a clear rationale.

The ongoing challenge for us all is to keep up to date with this knowledge, as both science and healthcare practice develops. Perhaps also, as your knowledge and competence develops, you will move knowledge and practice forward as well.

FURTHER READING

- James J, Baker C and Swain H (2002) *Principles of Science for Nurses*. Blackwell, Oxford. This book contains 14 chapters (252 pages) that link scientific principles to areas of common clinical practice. It is very readable and engaging. The chapters make extensive use of good diagrams to help readers to understand the topic area. A number of activities may be used by readers to develop ideas and to encourage participation within the text.
- Cree L and Rischmiller S (2001) *Science in Nursing* (4e). Harcourt, London. A large textbook (461 pages) that focuses on a broad range of scientific principles. Each chapter has a clear patient focus and is written in a no-nonsense and informative manner. This book will be a useful reference source over a long period of time. Readers do, however, need to be attentive and concentrate when reading this.
- Ross JS and Wilson KW (2002) *Anatomy and Physiology in Health and Illness* (9e). Churchill Livingstone, London. A good basic anatomy and physiology book that will serve you well. It is easy to read and has very good illustrations throughout. This text will be useful to anyone studying healthcare topics.

APPENDIX I

ANSWERS TO ACTIVITIES

Heat and metabolic rate
- Shivering, the rapid contraction of skeletal muscles, generates heat.
- Body hairs trap a layer of air. This air acts as an insulator reducing heat loss.
- Increased production of thyroxin by the thyroid gland. This increases the rate of cellular metabolism.
- Exercise.
- Vasoconstriction, the reduction of blood to the extremities of the body.

Heat energy
- Protein   17 kJ
- Carbohydrate   16 kJ
- Fat   37 kJ
- Alcohol   29 kJ

Temperature readings
You may have discovered that there is a variation of information related to this activity. This is because a range of values may be observed between healthy people. The body's temperature also varies depending on where the measurement is taken, the time of day, the influence of hormones (for example, the menstrual cycle), the environment, the emotional state of the individual, exercise or possible infection.

- Peripheral temperature = 36.6–37.0° Celsius (°C)
- Core temperature = 37.2–37.6°C

Heat exchange
- *Conduction* – The process by which heat is transmitted through a substance (solid or liquid) or from one substance to another when they are in contact.
- *Convection* – The process of heat transfer, through conduction, can be speeded up by the movement of gases or liquids. A good example of this may be found within most homes (a radiator). As the air (atmosphere) heats up the air molecules become less dense and rise. As the air rises it is replaced by cooler air. The cooler air, in turn, absorbs heat from the radiator and the cycle continues.
- *Radiation* – This method of heat transfer does not rely on any other substance (such as the movement of molecules). Heat loss is in the form of infra-red

radiant energy (thermal energy). This energy is transmitted through space in the form of waves called 'electromagnetic waves'.

- *Evaporation* – The evaporation process involves a change of state of a liquid. The change process from a liquid to a vapour requires energy, in the form of heat. This energy comes from the body. As the liquid takes heat from the body the molecules speed up and eventually when hot enough change to a gas state (vapour) and the heat disperses into the air – cooling down the body.

Chapter 9

THE DEVELOPING ROLE OF HEALTHCARE ASSISTANTS

Gareth Owens

INTRODUCTION

Care assistants support registered nurses, midwives and other health professionals with the provision of patient care. In many organisations this role has changed considerably over the past ten years. The reasons for this include the following:

- changing needs of patients and the healthcare they require
- introduction of supernumerary status for pre-registration students
- removal of the Enrolled Nurse grade
- difficulty of retaining sufficient numbers of registered staff.

As a consequence, many departments have enlarged the role of support workers to include work that was traditionally carried out solely by registered staff. For example, monitoring blood glucose, urinalysis, venepuncture and recording a 12-lead ECG. Developing staff to work across traditional boundaries in this way has allowed greater flexibility of care provision and provided benefits for both patients and staff. It has also produced a more challenging role for care assistants – one that requires increased competence, knowledge and responsibility.

This chapter explores how any enlargements to your role may be organised effectively – both by you and by your manager. It examines the principles of accountability and competence and how these relate to the legal requirement for you to provide safe patient care. Lastly, it proposes the adoption of a standardised code of conduct for support workers.

 Many of the proposals discussed in this chapter require the agreement and involvement of line managers. You should discuss their potential implementation either with them or with your team leaders.

THE CONSEQUENCES OF ROLE EXPANSION

We hope that you have found that taking on new and challenging activities has added to your enjoyment of work and has led to a more fulfilling career. However, you may also feel that adjusting to this expanded role has caused a certain amount of uncertainty and frustration; not only for you but also for the registered staff with whom you work. Before looking at some of the ways that role developments may be managed to reduce uncertainties, it will be useful to review your personal experience of these changes. Please complete the following activity and then compare your comments with those in Appendix I.

 Expanding the role of support workers

Think about how your role has changed as a result of taking on activities that were previously carried out by registered staff. If your role has remained unchanged, you will need to speculate about the consequences of taking on these extra responsibilities.

In one column make a list that identifies the advantages or opportunities that these changes will bring you and patients.

In another column record any disadvantages or concerns you may have about taking on these extra activities.

Principles for the Safe and Effective Delegation of Clinical Activity to Support Workers

You may find that many registered staff do not fully understand how to organise the activities carried out by support workers safely. Although standards and advice do exist, these are rather brief and fragmented statements that often lead to misinterpretation and uncertainty. We have condensed this advice into four principles that provide clear guidance to managers on how work can be delegated to you safely and effectively. They incorporate the guidance on this subject published by the Royal College of Nursing (RCN, 1991), the Department of Health (DoH, 1999) and the Nursing and Midwifery Council (NMC, 2002). Although these guidelines focus on enlargements to your role, they may also be applied in general terms to all the activities that you carry out.

Principles for the safe and effective delegation of clinical activity to support workers

- The role and responsibility of support workers must be clearly defined.
- Support workers must work under the direction of a registered practitioner who is accountable for the appropriate delegation and supervision of work.
- Support workers must be competent to undertake the work that is delegated to them and must never work beyond their level of competence.
- The implementation and outcome of all developments in the role of support workers must be monitored and evaluated.

Now let us look at these principles in more detail.

The Role and Responsibility of Support Workers Must Be Clearly Defined

All developments in your role must be based on a thorough assessment of patient need and should be introduced primarily in the interests of improving the care provided by your department – rather than, for example, just to reduce the costs of healthcare. You should be included in any discussions about proposed changes to your role and asked your opinion about the appropriateness of delegating extra responsibilities to you.

When asked to take on extra duties (especially those that were previously carried out by registered staff), you may have found that the extent and limits of these additional responsibilities were not explained clearly. At best this would have caused you some uncertainty and at worst could have resulted in unsafe practice if you had misinterpreted what was asked of you. For this reason, your extra responsibilities (and the limits of these) must be clearly stated and understood not only by you but also by all members of the team. In the case of simple wound dressings, for example, it would be necessary to have the rather broad term 'simple wound' described as follows:

> Support workers may only undertake simple wound dressings as agreed with a registered practitioner. Simple wounds are defined, according to the wound care guidelines, as either: (a) epithelialising, superficial or with low exudate; (b) granulating; or (c) moderately exuding. A registered practitioner should dress the following: those that are exuding copiously, yellow sloughy, malodorous, black/brown necrotic, cavity or bleeding.

Usually though, the definition of a new role need not be as detailed as this and may be addressed in a much shorter statement. But remember, if you are unsure about the extent and limits of your responsibility, you have a right to ask for clarification. Indeed, registered staff should actively encourage you to question their delegation in this way, as this will ensure that the care they ask you to deliver on their behalf remains safe and beneficial to patients.

SUPPORT WORKERS MUST WORK UNDER THE DIRECTION OF A REGISTERED PRACTITIONER WHO IS ACCOUNTABLE FOR THE APPROPRIATE DELEGATION AND SUPERVISION OF WORK

In other words, registered staff are accountable for the work they assign to you, so do not work independently of them. Instead, unless the way forward is obvious, keep your team leader up to date with all aspects of the care you deliver.

To be accountable is to accept responsibility for something or someone. It is often linked to the term 'answerability', which means being able to justify why a particular course of action was taken. In common terms this means that if you are accountable, 'the buck stops with you'. Unfortunately, when it comes to delegating work to care assistants, many registered staff are confused about who is accountable for the care that is delivered. They are not sure if they are responsible for an activity (because they have asked you to do it) or if you are (because it was you who actually carried it out). For this reason, you may find that some staff are unwilling to delegate particular activities to you – even though others, with a clearer understanding of accountability, may be confident to do so.

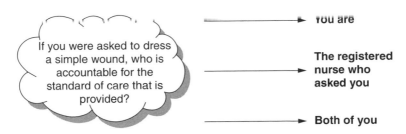

If you were asked to dress a simple wound, who is accountable for the standard of care that is provided?

You are

The registered nurse who asked you

Both of you

Figure 9.1 Who is accountable?

You may also share this uncertainty about accountability. For instance, if you were asked the question in Figure 9.1 how would you reply?

The answer, as you probably suspected, is both of you – but for different reasons. This is because support workers and registered practitioners are accountable to separate authorities.

Registered practitioners are accountable to their regulatory body (that is, *professionally accountable*) – for nurses, this would be to the Nursing and Midwifery Council (NMC) and for other professions, the Health Professions Council (HPC).

Because care assistants are not registered at present, you are not answerable to a regulatory body, but remain responsible to wider society (that is, *legally accountable*). Registered practitioners are also legally accountable.

Both of you are also *accountable to your employer*.

Now let us look at these three areas of accountability in more detail.

Professional accountability

The professional regulatory bodies hold registered practitioners accountable, both for their own practice and for ensuring that it is appropriate to delegate an activity to a support worker. For example, the NMC informs registered practitioners that:

> you may be expected to delegate care delivery to others who are not registered nurses or midwives . . . You remain *accountable for the appropriateness of the delegation*, for ensuring that the person who does the work is able to do it and that adequate supervision or support is provided.
>
> (NMC, 2002, p.7)

This means, in the example above, that registered practitioners are required to demonstrate to their regulatory body that it was appropriate to ask you to dress the wound; that is, that they were sure you were competent to carry out this particular procedure and that they had monitored your practice satisfactorily. If their actions in this respect were satisfactory, they would not be criticised for the outcomes of the care you had provided. As you are not a registered practitioner, the NMC or HPC will leave the question of your possible carelessness to the law or to your employer.

Legal accountability and accountability to your employer
However, this does not mean that responsibility for healthcare provision is restricted to registered staff. Indeed, two other authorities – the law and your employer – may hold you accountable for your actions and expect you to demonstrate that you performed the wound dressing competently. Furthermore, if you were judged to have acted inappropriately, you could be considered negligent in law and/or be disciplined by your employer.

So, both staff are accountable for their actions:

- registered practitioners for the appropriateness of their delegation to you
- you for ensuring that you carry out your work at a competent level.

SUPPORT WORKERS MUST BE COMPETENT TO UNDERTAKE THE WORK THAT IS DELEGATED TO THEM AND MUST NEVER WORK BEYOND THEIR LEVEL OF COMPETENCE

The issue of competence is vital: registered staff must be satisfied that you are competent to undertake an activity and you must accept this activity only if you are confident that you are able to carry it out to the required standard. However, you may find it is not always easy to describe what competence means or even to recognise it in yourself.

 Knowing your competence

Explain what the term competence means to you by completing the following statement.

Competence is

Think about how you would assure someone that you are competent to carry out a particular skill and then complete the following statement.

I am competent because

Competence

To be competent means to possess the skills and knowledge required for lawful, safe and effective practice. The law itself describes competence as carrying out an activity to the required standard – which prompts the question, 'What is the required standard?'. Helpfully, this was answered in the case of Bolam *v* Friern Hospital Management Committee (1957) with the following statement: 'The standard expected is the standard of the ordinary skilled person who carries out that skill'.

In other words, you do not have to achieve the highest expert skill to be considered competent; it is sufficient to practise at the average or usual level. This is a useful definition to bear in mind – whenever you are unsure of your competence to undertake a particular activity, ask yourself, 'Can I perform this skill to the same level as the people who usually carry it out?'. For example, if asked to monitor blood pressure, could you do this to the same level of skill and knowledge as a registered practitioner? If you can confidently answer yes and are able to support this conclusion, you should expect to be able to perform this skill safely and effectively.

Demonstration of competence

If you are asked to demonstrate that you have achieved a competent level of skill it will be helpful to be able to:

- explain how you initially learnt the skill and describe the amount and range of supervised practice that you undertook – *learning*
- show that you have had your knowledge and abilities assessed by a competent person – *assessment*
- explain how you have kept your knowledge and skill up to date with current practice – *maintenance*.

One of the benefits of undertaking an accredited vocational qualification, such as a National Vocational Qualification or Open College Network Programme, is that these three steps are an essential component of their assessment structure.

 If you are developing a new skill, but are not registered for an externally accredited qualification, it is a good habit to make brief notes that show you have undertaken the above three stages of learning, assessment and maintenance of competence. These notes could then be used as a record of how you achieved the required level of competence in that skill.

Similarly, managers should follow a similar process of facilitating and demonstrating the attainment of competence when they organise 'in-house' training programmes for support workers. For this reason, the following components of any learning programmes which have been developed 'in-house' should be documented and kept by your manager.

- A description of the clinical activity and the limits within which it is to be performed.
- The competencies required to carry out an activity, in terms of knowledge, skills and attitude. It may also be useful to describe competence in terms of a clinical protocol. If so, this should contain a list of the equipment required, followed by a step-by-step account of the procedure with an accompanying rationale for the actions described.
- A brief summary of how the learning has been organised, facilitated and assessed.
- A record that the support worker has been assessed as competent and is confident to practice. This should be signed and dated by the assessor and care assistant.

Even when you have undertaken a comprehensive training programme, if you feel unprepared for your new role, it is important that you acknowledge the limits of your competence and decline all duties that you cannot perform in a safe and skilled manner. Again, you will be encouraged and supported to do this by the registered staff with whom you work.

THE IMPLEMENTATION AND OUTCOME OF ALL DEVELOPMENTS IN THE ROLE OF SUPPORT WORKERS MUST BE MONITORED AND EVALUATED

The role development of care assistants must be properly supported and evaluated and, when required, adjustments made to minimise risks and maximise benefits. You will, therefore, be expected to contribute to an evaluation of the healthcare that has been delivered to patients as a result of your extra duties. When doing this, all developments in your role should be measured primarily in terms of patient safety and the effectiveness of the care provided. Your comments on this will be an important part of any changes that may need to be implemented.

A CODE OF CONDUCT FOR SUPPORT WORKERS

Most organisations for which you work will aim to provide you with a rewarding career and opportunities that help you to achieve your full potential. In return, they will expect you to undertake your work in a safe, skilled and *principled* manner.

Registered nurses, midwives and allied health professionals have these principles of correct behaviour identified in their codes of professional conduct. These are very helpful documents, as they contain clear information about the behaviour that is expected from all those who work in a particular profession. In general terms, all these codes require their members to act in ways that:

- protect and promote the interests of patients
- promote a constructive and collaborative working relationship with all members of the healthcare team
- justify public trust and confidence
- maintain the good standing and reputation of the organisation for which they work.

Unfortunately, there is no similar code of conduct for support workers. This is because, at present, you are not registered with a professional body or required by law to hold a recognised qualification. This is unfortunate, as many of the concerns and uncertainties that sometimes arise when taking on a wider role in healthcare could be resolved or prevented by clearer guidance on correct 'professional' behaviour.

 Principles of conduct

In the absence of a national code of conduct for support workers, it would be helpful to identify what you feel should be included in such a document. For example, you may believe it is important to make a statement about the importance of maintaining the confidentiality of patient information or that the dignity and self-esteem of patients should be protected.

Write down your thoughts and feelings about what constitutes correct behaviour and attitude in your current job role.

Compare your ideas with the statements contained within a code of conduct*
that has been adopted by the support workers of one NHS Trust (Box 9.1).

* Acknowledgement: Sections of these principles are based upon the *NMC*
Code of Professional Conduct (NMC, 2002).

Box 9.1   Code of Conduct for support workers

The following *Code of Conduct* identifies the standards of behaviour and
attitude that are required of all support workers who work within the Trust.
You should use these principles to ensure that the care you provide is of the
highest possible standard.

1   Always act under the direction and supervision of a registered practitioner.

   *This is because the regulatory bodies of Nursing and Midwifery and the Allied Health
   Professions regard the registered practitioner that you work with as being* **professionally**
   responsible for the results of your actions and for delegating work to you.

2   Carry out all activities safely, effectively and to the best of your abilities,
   in accordance with the policies and protocols of the Trust.

   *This is because, although registered practitioners are professionally responsible for the
   results of your actions, you remain accountable for them in* **law** *and also to the* **Trust** *that
   employs you.*

3   Do not take on an activity unless you can carry it out safely and
   effectively.

4   If you do not feel ready to take on an activity, report this to a registered
   practitioner and ask them to help you develop the knowledge and skills
   that you need.

5   Work in partnership with patients and, whenever possible, support their
   rights to choice, independence and self-management.

6   Promote and maintain the dignity and privacy of patients.

7   Respect the individuality and diversity of patients and do not discriminate
   against them in any way.

8 Treat information about patients as confidential; disclose this information only when patients give their permission, when you are required to do so by law or when it is justified in the public interest.

9 If the care required by a patient conflicts with your moral beliefs, report this to a registered practitioner and continue the necessary care until the appropriate course of action has been agreed.

10 Do not abuse the trust that patients place in you: always protect and promote their interests and make sure that all aspects of your relationship with them are determined solely by their healthcare needs.

11 Do not accept gifts or favours that may influence the care that you give or might be interpreted by others as an attempt to influence you.

12 Work constructively with all members of the healthcare team: respect their skills, value their contributions and professional judgement, treat them fairly and do not discriminate against them in any way.

© Oxford Radcliffe Hospitals NHS Trust, 2002

FINAL THOUGHTS

In recent years, you may have found that your role has expanded to include work that was carried out mostly by registered staff in the past. Although this role expansion will have provided you with a more challenging and fulfilling career, it may also have led to a certain amount of frustration and uncertainty. Fortunately, understanding the implications of personal accountability and competence, combined with clear principles for delegating work to care assistants, will reduce these uncertainties and so help to ensure you can accept these extra responsibilities with confidence and enthusiasm.

REFERENCES

DoH (1999) *Making a Difference. Strengthening the Nursing, Midwifery and Health Visiting Contribution to Health Care*. Department of Health, London.

NMC (2002) *Code of Professional Conduct*. Nursing and Midwifery Council, London.

RCN (1991) *The Role of the Support Worker within the Professional Nursing Team*. Issues in Nursing and Health No. 15. Royal College of Nursing, London.

APPENDIX 1

EXPANDING THE ROLE OF SUPPORT WORKERS

These answers were compiled following a discussion with 16 nursing healthcare assistants from an acute NHS Trust who had recently experienced changes to their role. The comments, although derived from nursing, probably also relate to the experiences of a wide range of support workers and other allied healthcare professions.

Advantages/opportunities

- It has made my job more interesting.
- The patients get things done more quickly – the nurses are too busy to do everything themselves.
- We are with the patients all the time, so it makes sense that we take on more things rather than get the nurses to do them.
- It makes me think about my job more.
- I understand why things are done now – before I would tend to just do them because I was told to.
- It has encouraged me to apply for other courses and think about training to be a nurse.

Disadvantages/concerns

- There is no consistency among the nurses – some are confident to let me do the things I was trained to do, whereas others are not and say it is a trained nurse's role.
- The nurses will not let me do some things, because they do not want to be responsible for anything that might go wrong.
- It is interesting to do extra things, but it is 'cheap labour' – we should be paid more for taking on extra roles.
- I am willing to take on more, but I am not always sure what I am allowed to do and what I should leave to the nurses.
- I am not sure who is 'covering me' if something goes wrong.

INDEX